What Readers Are Saying

— • • —

"In *Yes, You Can Heal*, Diane Goldner expertly guides the reader to discover his or her own magical abilities to heal. As Diane shares real-life examples of some of the hundreds of people she has worked with, it is clear that she is not only a gifted healer, she is also a gifted teacher. This book is a must-read for healers, anyone trying to heal an illness or a chronic condition, or for anyone who wishes to heal an aspect of his or her life that is out of balance, or is in need of greater harmony and vitality."

—JULIE HOYLE, author of *An Awakened Life*

"I devoured this book in one bite. *Yes, You Can Heal* is a light-hearted yet deeply meaningful book about how to tap into the soul of personal healing. Like Diane's first book, *How People Heal*—which was a profound balm for my personal healing and led me on my path to become a healer—this book radiates light and feels divinely guided."

—REV. LISA MILLER, host of *Women's Well* Radio Show, Lexington, KY

"For the individual looking to heal, Diane's book will be their encyclopedia. I found it incredible. Each and every sentence packs a wallop. She shares undeniable truths and tools to trans-form and create health, on all levels. No one is left in the dark and helpless. I'm absolutely blown away by the insights found in *Yes, You Can Heal*."

—LYNN FALKOWSKI, R.N., retired operating room nurse

"Diane Goldner has been a part of my family's life for over ten years. My wife and I have a daughter who has multiple medical issues including 15 major spinal surgeries, optic gliomas, bone infections and dozens of hospitalizations.

Over the years I have seen Diane's energy healing have a deep and profound effect on virtually every member of our family. I have seen nerve inflammation reduced, tumors shrink, anxiety relieved, PTSD managed and spines straightened.

At my daughter's last doctor's appointment the oncologist was so pleased to see her optic tumors had become completely inactive. He remarked, 'I don't know what you're doing, but keep it up.' This was after multiple MRIs and healings with Diane.

Through the years as I came to rely on Diane's healing energy she would always insist that her skills and gifts were not exclusive to her. Now, in *Yes, You Can Heal,* Diane teaches us how to make healing our own gift to ourselves, and the world."

—JERRY RUSTALIA, R.N.

"I stumbled upon *How People Heal* several years ago and was amazed with how Diane Goldner brilliantly explained the somewhat esoteric topic of healing. It was my "go to" for anyone curious or skeptical about energy healing or the mind-body-spirit connection.

Now with *Yes, You Can Heal,* Diane goes to the specific. We all have the power to heal ourselves, but how? Think of *Yes, You Can Heal* as a comprehensive owner's manual, an easy-to-follow guide for anyone looking to feel, get and be better. There is so much great stuff!"

—MARA LANDIS, founder of NutmegAspirin.com

"Thank you, Diane, for sharing your vast knowledge of subtle energy healing in this unique book. Through your gifts as a healer and teacher I have personally experienced a transformation that restored me to health, and enhanced my spiritual practice and my work as a therapist. Your wisdom and spirit empowers *Yes, You Can Heal*. I highly recommend this book."

—ROBERT BORESS, LMFT

"Diane Goldner gives us uplifting and life-changing lessons in how to heal your body and your life. Her sparkling gifts as a writer, healer and teacher make this book a joy to read."

—KAREN CAMPBELL, clairvoyant

"I was so deeply impacted by Diane's wisdom about energy healing in *Yes, You Can Heal,* including the power of the ways she shares that we can use to heal ourselves. At a time when chronic illness has reached epidemic proportions, this is a much-needed book. Reading it, I experienced the deep truth of its pure and uplifting energy."

—ROBERT UGRASENA KEMTER, Awaken the Dreamer Facilitator, Panchamama Alliance and former manager, SYDA Foundation

"Diane has done it again. In *Yes, You Can Heal* Diane shares the fascinating and enlightening world of energy healing in an understandable and down-to-earth way, even for those with no background in this field. Diane has gifted us once more with her talents as a healer, teacher and author."

—NANCY REUBEN, M.D., physician, healer and author of *Self-Care & Self-Empowerment Through Energy Awareness* CD Series

Yes, You Can Heal

THE SECRET TO TRANSFORMING ILLNESS AND CREATING A RADIANT LIFE

DIANE GOLDNER

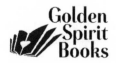

Golden Spirit Books

NEW YORK • LOS ANGELES

Golden Spirit Books
P.O. Box 581
Santa Monica, CA 90406
GoldenSpiritBks@gmail.com

First Golden Spirit Books edition 2018

A portion of the proceeds from *Yes, You Can Heal* will be donated to charities dedicated to the upliftment of people.

For information about special bulk purchases, contact:
Golden Spirit Books at 310-264-1924
or GoldenSpiritBks@gmail.com.

Cover and Interior Design: Amy Gingery
Photograph of Diane: Jeff Fasano
Library of Congress Control Number: 2017902455
ISBN #978-1-940044-02-6

This book should not take the place of personalized medical care or treatment. This book contains the opinions and ideas of its author and is intended to provide useful information on its subject matter. It is sold with the understanding that the author and publisher are not engaged in rendering professional services via this book. The author and publisher disclaim all liability in connection with the use of this book.

It is that Perfect Power alone that heals;
all external methods of stimulation only cooperate with
the life energy and are valueless without it.

—PARAMAHANSA YOGANANDA
Scientific Healing Affirmations

Table of Contents

————— • • • —————

Guided Meditations

——— • • ———

Foreword

───── • • • ─────

BY ALLISON DUBOIS

"Figuring out our gifts in life is part of our journey to becoming enlightened human beings."

P eople have considered Diane Goldner a world-class healer for years, and I've seen it firsthand.

A friend of mine, Michele, had an aggressive form of cancer. She and her husband, her college sweetheart, had two young daughters. It was painful to watch their family go through such a frightening and devastating experience.

I called Diane to ask her for her help. I'm a medium and I deal with the dead; she deals with the living and, sometimes, the dying. I was hoping that Diane could buy my friend a little more time with her daughters. I have three daughters of my own and I couldn't imagine leaving them at such a young age.

Michele was at death's door, but after her session with Diane she miraculously went into remission. Michele was able to spend four more years with her girls. The oldest was a senior in high school when her mother died—still so very young, but better equipped to understand death.

The girls had four additional years of happy memories with their mother. We were all so grateful for the extra time we had with Michele, and there's no doubt in my mind that it was Diane who made those years possible.

For more than a decade, I've recommended Diane as a healer. Now in *Yes, You Can Heal*, Diane shows you how to connect with your own deepest wisdom and light, and shares the secrets of healing with you. There is no better gift than that.

—ALLISON DUBOIS is the inspiration behind the hit TV show *Medium*, *New York Times* bestselling author of *Don't Kiss Them Good-Bye* and *We Are Their Heaven*, and a weekly columnist for Australia's *New Idea* magazine.

Introduction

———— • • • ————

FROM SKEPTIC TO HEALER

I f you are reading this, there is probably something you would like to heal. My goal in writing this book is to help you heal deeply. You can begin to move immediately from pain or illness to radiant health and joy.

When I started exploring energy healing, I was a curious, but highly skeptical journalist. For me it all began when the founder of a charity I had interviewed for *The New York Times* brought me to meet her spiritual teacher, a meditation master from India who was said to have special powers to transform my life. At the time I was sure I had wasted my day, but later I would feel quite differently.

Soon after that encounter, a doctor showed me a book on energy healing. I had gone to an Ivy League school, Barnard College at Columbia University, and as a journalist I read as many as four newspapers a day. I considered myself well informed. Yet I had never heard of this type of healing. It seemed hard to believe it could be real. But what if it was? I decided that I would investigate to get to the bottom of these claims.

I began an intensive study of healing for a magazine assignment. As I did my research, I discovered that energy healing got results. I was more than a little unnerved. The power of these subtle energies seemed revolutionary. Yet, ultimately it was so logical and so effective. Why weren't these techniques widely used?

How did this type of healing really work? I wondered. What did the scientific record say? I wanted answers to these questions. Thus, the magazine article turned into a five-year investigation that led to my first book, *Infinite Grace: Where the Worlds of Science and Spiritual Healing Meet* (reissued in paperback as *How People Heal*).

Those five years turned my world inside out. My understanding of health, and even the very nature of reality, changed dramatically. My idea of what we humans are capable of also changed.

Every time a healer I interviewed told me about a technique they used, I would think to myself: *This can't be true.* So I would try it, simply to prove to myself that it indeed was just so much hype. It would always work. Indeed, this type of healing seemed so easy. At the same time, all of my subtle and spiritual energies— energies that I hadn't known existed—were awakening.

Early on, for instance, I worked with an acquaintance suffering from a chronic Candida infection in her gut. As soon as I started my first healing, I could see the underlying energies that were allowing this invasion to overtake her digestive system. I worked hard to transmute them. When the session was over I left her house. Minutes later I was overcome by the most powerful desire to eat cake. It was as if I was possessed. I knew then just how anguished she felt. But after only two healings that overwhelming urge was gone from her system. Her cravings stopped, and she was able to stay on her diet.

In such a way, I did many healings and received many more healings in the process of trying to understand what, exactly, is subtle energy and how it can be used for healing. I soon discovered that I could do this kind of healing even long distance. I would be able to touch into another person's energy, and know things that they themselves didn't know, and clear issues for them, as if they were right there in the room with me.

I was quite fortunate to be mentored by the most gifted healers teaching at that time, including Rosalyn Bruyere, Kabbalist Jason Shulman, Amy Skezas, and Barbara Brennan and several of her students, and studied the Light Body teachings of Luminessence founders Sanaya Roman and Duane Packer. I also talked to the leading scientists and medical doctors investigating this area, including researchers at the University of Arizona Medical School and physicists at Princeton University. I could see how the science and spirituality were related; indeed, in some ways, they were simply different ways of talking about the same thing.

Infinite Grace was finally published in 1999 (now *How People Heal*) with explorations of the scientific studies on healing and the experiences of healers and those they healed. I expected to go back into journalism. But it was not to be. People kept asking me for healings, and eventually I had to accept that I had a new and deeper calling. (I share my process of transformation in my memoir of becoming a healer, *Awakening to the Light*.)

I've been a healer now for twenty years. I've worked with thousands of people facing just about any kind of issue you can imagine, including anxiety, chronic illness, infertility, cancer, trauma and surgery. I've also helped people with life challenges such as resolving money issues, improving relationships, creating good boundaries, and recovering true self-esteem.

I've worked with many different types of people from all walks of life. Some tell me they might not typically seek out a healer. Still, I've always been surprised by how open most people are spiritually. I've helped doctors, nurses, mothers and fathers, babies, CEOs, even an Olympic athlete who was injured on the eve of the games but went on to win several medals after just two healings.

Daily I read in the news or hear about people who could be helped by energy healing—if only they knew that it existed. I always wish I could reach out to them. That is why I am writing this book: to reach out to you and share with you so that you can heal.

Mehmet Oz, M.D., a renowned heart surgeon and the host of *The Dr. Oz Show,* whom I interviewed for my first book, called energy medicine "the next big frontier in medicine" in 2007 while on *Oprah.* I, too, have faith that science will eventually catch up with the mystics. There is already strong research in this area, including double blind studies, which I explore in my first book, *How People Heal.*

Most Western medicine is still currently based on simple biochemistry. It is rooted in the Newtonian paradigm, where everything in the universe is made of separate things. The subtle energy that we use in healing works in the quantum domain, where physicists have documented an underlying oneness in the universe.

As a healer, I have seen many small and large "miracles" take place. The healings only *seem* miraculous. When you understand and apply the principles of energy medicine, these healings are completely logical. By analogy, just imagine how magical a TV or smartphone would seem to someone from the 19th century. For this reason I think of energy healing as 25th century medicine. But it is available to you right now.

The practices I share with you in this book go far beyond simply telling you what's wrong. You can literally change your energy so your body is healed and your life takes on more radiance and ease.

Some types of pain, injury and illness can even go away almost immediately. For instance:

> Peter was gripped with sudden, but excruciating back pain. His whole back was seized up and he was practically immobile. When we started the healing, I ran high frequencies for illumination and flow. Soon, Peter knew the cause: the anger he had repressed in response to his critical mother-in-law. He had tried to help her put her house in order over the weekend. She had been anything but grateful. With this insight, he relaxed. He no longer had

4

to bottle up the anger and express it through his body. By the next morning the pain was totally gone.

• • •

Ilana had suffered from irritable bowel syndrome for fifteen years. For the past eight years it had been crippling. She couldn't leave the house to walk her daughter three blocks to school without worrying about an attack that would require a bathroom immediately. She was on two anti-anxiety medicines and lived on imodium pills. By the time she came to me for a healing, she recalled, "I was at my wit's end."

During the first session, I ran energy into her stomach and bowels. "I immediately felt calmer," she told me later. "After that session, I never had that unrest in my stomach again that always preceded an attack." After the second session, she dropped all of her medicine. After about five sessions, her irritable bowel syndrome was gone.

"I had tried everything," Ilana said. "Medicine, colonoscopies, blood tests, food allergy tests, acupuncture, psychiatry. The only thing that worked was you. You have absolutely changed my life."

• • •

As a teenager, Marilyn had a motorcycle accident that left her with a leg injury that required 60 stitches. Her doctors had feared she would ultimately lose her leg.

Every day she visualized the immune system working on her wound and radiant light going through it. "I don't know what made me do that," she told me years later, when I interviewed her as a scientist studying energy healing and consciousness. But Marilyn's healing methods worked.

Her leg healed completely. She was so inspired that she went on to study the mind-body connection as a research scientist, helping to bring scientific understanding of healing and consciousness to the world.

• • •

When Stacy called me for a healing, she was undergoing radiation treatment for breast cancer. Her upper body was covered in second and third degree burns. The burns were blistering and wrapped from the front to the back of her body. She was desperate for relief. She was on the east coast and I was in Los Angeles so I did a long distance healing.

The following morning, the blistering burns had "shrunk up," she recalls. "It was more like a rash than a burn. It was a miracle. You couldn't use another word to describe it. I'm an M.I.T.-trained physicist. That was proof to me that energy healing works. I should have taken pictures to show the doctors."

• • •

Andrew had a migraine headache, the type that would normally last for days or even a week. His blood pressure had also skyrocketed. As I tuned in for a long distance healing, I could tell he was feeling completely overwhelmed. He had put a lot of pressure on himself to achieve certain things at his company, where he was the CEO. That pressure was compressing his entire energy field. I slowly got all of his energy to flow and his breathing to expand and flow as well. The next morning his blood pressure was back to normal, the headache was gone and he woke feeling enthusiastic about life once again.

• • •

Bethany was in pain from a kidney stone. During a healing session, we got in touch with the fear that she had been holding in her body since childhood. As I ran energy, waves and waves of fear came up. As each wave arose, I held light to transmute the fear and bring in divine love.

Eventually the waves of fear subsided. I knew a shift had been made. For the next twenty-four hours, Bethany had excruciating pain. I suspected the kidney stone might be dissolving and told her to hang in. A day later she was feeling great. She called me a week later, after she had a new x-ray. "You won't believe it," she told me. "The kidney stone is gone. The technician reading the scan was amazed."

• • •

When Catherine, who had studied energy healing with me, learned that her blood sugar was off the charts and she had diabetes, the doctors cautioned her she would most likely get worse. She realized immediately that if she wanted to heal she would have to take matters into her own hands.

She said the diabetes diagnosis inspired her to implement everything she had learned about healing in her studies with me. "I had a life-threatening disease. I decided I'm not going to put up with this. I'm going to tackle it. It was a new emotional space for me that I developed studying energy skills with you," she told me. "In the past, my pattern would have been helplessness, and to be shocked and feel lost."

She knew from studying healing that the body was simply the most obvious expression of a number of other, more subtle levels, and that healing was possible. She did research and found a diet that she felt strongly would work for her to reverse her diabetes. It required the correct balance of complex carbohydrates, fat and protein, including never eating carbohydrates without protein. In just five months, she lost 34 pounds and brought her blood sugar levels down to normal.

Then, when a study came out announcing that the contestants on the TV show *The Biggest Loser* had trouble keeping weight off after their diet success, she worried, "How am I going to keep this weight off?" The answer came in a dream where she was with a very overweight woman with whom she used to work.

The woman told her she was losing weight with a very simple method: "I imagine these little balls of energy in my fat cells. And they make my fat cells soften and then they dissolve." Catherine said she began using that technique in her meditation the very next day.

"This is the time to work on everything in a higher, more beautiful, liberating level," said Catherine. "I had a breakthrough into a whole different realm." She told me that by teaching her to work in the subtle realms, "You changed my life. Maybe you saved it."

Whatever you would like to heal, use this book as a companion, day and night, whenever you want support, healing light or guidance. Even if you've been searching for help for a long time, don't give up. Help is truly available to you. You can even heal chronic conditions over time, and you will also uplift your entire life.

The techniques I am going to share with you are surprisingly simple. But I have found them to be profound and I hope you will too. Many of these techniques come from the *Vedas*, the earliest sacred texts of India; the Judeo-Christian wisdom of the Kabbalah; the healing teachers and Indian meditation masters with whom I have studied; and other esoteric sources that have been tested over millennia and passed down from one practitioner to another, and from master to student.

Everything I share has been helpful to me and to the people who have come to me for healings. When I first began my healing journey, I would try different ways of working with the energy and my consciousness. I would just see what worked for me. So I invite you to explore in whatever way suits you. At the same time, continue to work with the healing practitioners to whom you feel drawn. While it is essential to go within to heal and shift your energy, it also helps during a deep healing process to have support from others, as well.

I include many stories of healings in this book as a way of sharing how the healing process works. I hope reading about these healings gives you insights that will help you.

You can read the book from start to finish. You may also want to jump ahead to take a look at Chapter 12: "Seven Essentials for Healing." Another way you can use this book is to hold it in your hand when you have a question, and see what page it naturally opens to. Perhaps you will find the guidance you need right there.

You can apply the healing tools in this book immediately. They are easy to implement, and will enhance everything else you do. I have found them to be the secret keys to transformation, and hope you do, too.

• • •

Author's Note: All of the healing examples in this book involve real people and their true stories. I have changed names and identifying information to protect privacy.

The exercises in this book are meant to be complementary to Western medicine. They are not a substitute for regular medical care. If you are having symptoms of any sort, please see a medical professional.

ONE

A Higher Perspective

—— • • • ——

WE COME HERE TO LEARN AND DEVELOP

You may be wondering why you are in pain or ill. From a spiritual perspective, it is never to punish you or make you suffer.

You come to this life to develop and progress, and you encounter experiences that help you to do so. Illnesses and physical challenges are part of this process. Indeed, whatever happens in your life is designed to have a beneficial purpose. Illness and other challenges can be extremely difficult, but they are designed to help you develop your soul light. At the core of your being you are already radiant and whole. There is a pure energy of grace and peace. This is the state you are being guided to access.

Even some of the great saints had physical challenges, and those who didn't suffer physical pain or illness still had challenges of one kind or another. Just as we have to engage in physical exercise to develop and sustain our muscles, we all have to exercise our soul qualities to bring them forward and be one with our soul light.

We don't cause our problems, as some people suggest. Most of us would not consciously choose a path that would lead to pain. But we all have lessons to learn to bring us into greater alignment with our soul or Higher Self. When you learn the lessons your soul

11

sets for you, your life naturally expands. Regardless of what difficulty is in your life, there is always hope. There is always light. There is always grace for you.

Everything that occurs in your life is designed to guide you toward greater illumination, meaning that you can develop or strengthen qualities such as gentleness, courage, patience, kindness, forgiveness, truth, insight, gratitude, compassion, self-love and centeredness.

You are always being guided to let go of constrictions in thinking and understanding. The very things we think of as difficulties are there to help us burnish our being, and more fully embody the wisdom and light of our Higher Self.

When you expand your consciousness, you live with more flow, ease and grace. This may mean physical healing, but it may also involve much more. How this works is something we'll be exploring from many different angles. It is almost impossible to imagine how free and easy you can feel until it happens. But it is worth everything to experience this grace.

THE PURPOSE OF PAIN

From a spiritual perspective, there is usually some higher purpose to pain. It is not there to punish you, but rather to free you, to wake you up, to move you forward toward the inner light—to evolve you toward becoming one with your soul. There's powerful truth in the seemingly glib phrase, *Everything happens for the best.* Just keeping this in mind can help you search for how this could possibly be true.

Whatever challenge you are facing, use it as a doorway to make your whole life better, more radiant. It's in the very places you're having difficulty that the opportunity for deep transformation exists.

Look at each challenge as a gift and be grateful. Once you open that gift by gaining insight and inner shifts, you will receive everything your soul or Higher Self wants to give you. The meaning of some gifts are apparent immediately, while other situations can take many years to understand, heal and transform. Don't give up, even if clarity doesn't come right away.

HEALING IS A JOY

Energy healing is profound. It can be fun. It is always engrossing. It can feel miraculous. It's a little like being released from whatever prison you've been in, whether it is emotional, physical, psychological, or involves fear, doubt or trauma.

Healing has to do with bringing your whole life to a "higher order" or "higher flow," terms I use frequently. To understand a higher order, think of an ordinary house compared with a house that is exciting and inspiring. The two may have the same square footage, but there is a special feeling in the exciting house that is reflected in every angle and in each moment.

For a higher flow, you might think of driving in the car pool lane versus being stuck in bumper-to-bumper traffic. When your energy is flowing, you have access to your inner wisdom and your vitality. Having a higher flow in your life can mean moving out of pain and having things unfold effortlessly. It can mean experiencing more harmony, more joy, more acceptance. It means moving out of the groove you've been stuck in.

Healing and curing aren't always synonymous. For some, healing may happen at the physical level immediately. At other times, for various reasons, healing occurs first on nonphysical levels. Sometimes it won't completely transfer to the physical plane—it might be about gaining a new perspective on life. It might even be about passing in a more free and conscious way. In any case, healing is about a state of being that is exciting and expansive.

You could say that healing is about connecting to the deepest light and wisdom within you. It's like lighting a candle to illuminate the darkness. When you connect to the source, when you bring in illumination, the constrictions naturally release. Darkness and pain dissolve.

The great news is that in the process of healing your body, you will create a higher path forward in your life. Your soul always wants the best for you; it is always guiding you, encouraging you toward greater light and greater expansion.

Any discomfort or illness in your body is one way in which your soul works to get your attention. In this book, I will show you how to communicate with your soul and receive this precious guidance directly.

It is hard to do all of our healing by ourselves; there is no question that good practitioners can help greatly. I highly recommend that you get all the help you can from others. Still, it is always beneficial to have tools you can turn to at any time, day or night. After all, you are always with yourself.

BODY & SOUL

The understanding that health is connected to the soul is an ancient one. One of the Latin words for healing is *cura*, meaning "spiritual charge of souls," and in Middle English the word cure meant, "care of souls." Another Latin word for healing is *sanitas*, which can also translate as "purity, sanity, soundness of body, and soundness of mind." The ancient Norse word for healing meant "holy" and "spiritual." The Hebrew word for healing, *rapha*, is closely related both to spiritual and physical redemption and to wholeness.

This connection between body and soul is very real. The mediating force is our subtle energy. What is that subtle energy? It took me years to understand. Now I can distill it for you quite succinctly:

Your subtle energy refers to everything about you that is nonphysical. This includes your life force or *chi*; emotions and thoughts; desires and intentions; beliefs and memories; and spiritual light.

These energies are very real. They are not so much subtle as fundamental and highly significant. For me, they are also quite tangible. They can become that way for you, too. You probably already notice certain energies in yourself and others. For instance, if someone is angry, you may find that you resonate with that energy. Or if someone is happy you may feel uplifted being in their presence.

As these energies move about the body they flow through specific channels (many of which are used in acupuncture) and are regulated by vortexes of energy, known in Sanskrit as chakras, with which energy healers often work. Ultimately these energies permeate every cell of your body and are involved in every experience in your life. (Take a look at Chapter 13: "Your Energy Anatomy" for more details on how it all fits together.)

In the same way we use our hands to touch or move a physical object, I use my energy to interact with energy. I use higher frequencies to transmute the denser energies that cause blocks and leaks, and I will show you how you can do this, too. You will be doing this, not as a technician, but as a budding master.

Take a look at the "14 Paths To Healing" on the next page to explore different ways to understand and experience healing light in your life.

YOUR ENERGY, YOUR LIFE

When you work with energy and light, you are working at a fundamental, causative level. Once you change the energy, the physical change typically follows. It's a little like resolving errors in a document by going into the computer file and changing the electronic template instead of scratching out the mistakes on the printed page. Or you can think of it as being like baking—just as it's easier to modify the taste and texture of a cake before you

14 Paths To Healing

1. Dissolving Pain

2. Creating Vitality

3. Clearing Limitations

4. Gaining New Insights

5. Changing Thoughts and Feelings
   That Don't Serve You

6. Connecting to Divine Source/
   Your Higher Self

7. Letting Go of Limiting Beliefs

8. Living Your Life More Fully

9. Experiencing More Peace and Joy

10. Having a Higher Perspective

11. Learning to Trust Your Intuition

12. Regaining Your Power

13. Acceptance and Surrender

14. Living with More Ease, Flow and Grace

• • •

set it by baking it in the oven, it is easier to make changes at the energy level than at the physical level.

Your subtle energy is the template for your body and your life. It is not a by-product of your body. Rather, your subtle energy is the essence of who you are. When you work at the subtle energy level, you can often accomplish more with less effort. This doesn't mean, though, that healing is always easy. Sometimes there is only one thing more difficult than healing, and that is not healing.

You may have to go deep within to find the issues underlying your pain, but some form of healing is always possible. Sometimes the answer may not seem evident. In that case, just work with adding light and energy. The light will always help. At the same time, set your intention for radiant health. (For more guidance on working at the level of intention, take a look at Chapter 12: "Seven Essentials for Healing.")

ASK FOR THE HIGHEST

If you are feeling an urgent need for healing right now, help is always there. Sometimes you just need the comfort and presence of light, of high frequencies of energy, a transmission of love. Try the guided meditation, "Ask for the Highest Healing," at the end of this chapter. You may experience some immediate relief. Even if you don't feel better in the moment, you will be guided on where to get the help that you need, often in the next day or two. The light knows what's best for you and will always help bring things to a higher order, whether or not you can completely perceive how it is working.

As you will see, in this meditation and elsewhere, I invite you to call in your Higher Self, the part of you that is all knowing and all loving. You may also bring in a spiritual master or angel, if you feel drawn to do so. Or simply focus on light and divine love. These meditations will work, whatever your beliefs. They are designed to help you explore your consciousness and expand your awareness.

I know firsthand that it may be difficult to believe in realms that most of us can't see. When first investigating healing, I was intrigued that some people could see into other realms, but also found it almost impossible to believe. When I mentioned this to Barbara Brennan, a healer originally trained as a physicist, she noted that just as there is a range of life from the gigantic to the microscopic, there is a range of life on the vibrational scale. At the time, I found that to be a comforting perspective.

Over time, as I opened up, I began to sense these other levels. Especially in the beginning, it always came as a surprise. Now that I have been a healer for many years, I can say that divine beings come more often than you would think to help us heal, whether we believe in them or not, or consciously experience them or not. For me, even now it is always a special event. I find that guidance generally comes in a form that has deep meaning for the person with whom I am working. I'll share one experience that exemplifies this.

Many years ago, a woman who was going through a divorce brought her pre-teen daughter in for a healing session. As I started the healing, I saw on my inner mind screen that the room was filled with angels. I had never seen angels before, except in illustrations and paintings.

Afterwards, I told the mother, "By the way, there were a lot of angels there for your daughter." She replied, "My daughter will be happy to hear that. She has been praying for days that all of her angels would be present for the healing."

You can always ask for help and you will receive it. Before you try the guided meditation, "Ask for the Highest Healing," you may want to take a look at "Creating a Sacred Space." You can refer back to this as you do the meditations in this book.

Creating a Sacred Space

For the meditations in this book, you may want to create a sacred space within which to work. This will help you go into a deeper state and feel safe as you meditate. Here are a few practices that have worked well for me:

* Make sure the room where you will meditate is clean and orderly.

* Make sure you will not be disturbed during meditation.

* You can light a candle and dedicate your meditation journey to the divine before you begin.

* Consider adding fresh flowers either before each meditation or weekly.

* If you wish, you can also set up an altar by putting a picture of a master, angel, god or goddess, or saint on a table. Or you can place a sacred book, such as a Bible or book of sutras, there. Or find a beautiful picture of nature for your altar, something that connects you to the beauty of all that is.

* For an even deeper experience, you can start any meditation in this book by going into Deep Relaxation in "Seven Essentials for Healing."

• • •

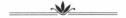

Ask for the Highest Healing

When you urgently need healing support, do this guided meditation. Trust that help is there. You may notice things shifting during the healing, or a few days later. For instance, you may feel relief or find you are guided to see a particular healing practitioner after you do this meditation.

1. Go into a state of Deep Relaxation. (Follow the instructions in Chapter 12: "Seven Essentials for Healing.")

2. Call in the light and divine love, and bring in your Higher Self. If you wish, you may also call in any healing masters or archangels to whom you feel drawn.

3. Imagine that you are in the healing room of a temple in a very high dimension. Everything is made of shimmering light.

4. See yourself lying on the healing table, which itself may be formed of light.

5. Imagine or see your Higher Self there with you, holding your feet and then placing hands on your heart, running the most beautiful divine light into you. If you've called in any masters or archangels see them also holding you and transmitting light and love to you.

6. Experience all the great love and compassion that is there for you.

7. As you lie on the table receiving healing light, allow yourself to go deeper and deeper into relaxation.

8. Stay here, receiving healing light and love, for as long as you want.

9. Feel the gratitude and love in your own heart for the help and love you are receiving.

10. When you are ready, thank the light and your Higher Self and any masters or archangels you called in. Gently come back to the room and come out of meditation.

You can do this meditation as often as you life. Help will always be there for you.

TWO

Your Body, Your Soul

————— • • • —————

THERE IS NOTHING ORDINARY ABOUT A HUMAN BODY
YOUR SOUL SPEAKS THROUGH YOUR BODY

When you have pain, it usually means there is something your soul, or higher self, wants you to know. When you take the time to tune in to your soul's message, you can begin to heal. Even though I have been offering healing light for many years, I still find it remarkable how much can shift, sometimes very quickly, simply through gaining more awareness of the soul issues underlying the physical pain.

Take Barbara's situation. When she came to see me, her hands had been atrophying for about six years. Her hands were so weak she couldn't open a jar. A pretty, dark-haired, delicate woman in her 50s, Barbara was happily married and generally content. So why, I wondered, were her hands failing her? "Did any major event occur in your life perhaps a year or two before your hands started to get weak?" I asked.

"Not really," Barbara said. Then, after reflecting for a moment, she lit up as if something she had always known had suddenly clicked into place. "Well, you know," she said, "My husband had a skydiving accident." She explained how she had watched him fall past the tree line without his parachute fully opening. His very survival was a miracle. She had taken care of him during the many months of his recovery from his injuries.

As Barbara relaxed on my healing table, I ran energy into her hands and heart. Soon her hands began to tell me their story: Barbara had come face-to-face with the possibility of her husband's death, and she simply couldn't *handle* it.

Silently, I transmitted to Barbara the message that I knew would help her heal: *Whatever happened, she had the inner strength to handle it, and she and her loved ones would always be held in God's hands.* I did this silently, soul to soul, through telepathic communication, because the message comes through then as a deep inner knowing.

Barbara's hands improved after the healing. But months later her elderly mother fell ill, and Barbara's hands took a turn for the worse. When Barbara came in for a second healing, I saw that she was again facing the one thing she felt she could not *handle*: the possible death of someone she loved. I ran a great deal of energy through her hands and strengthened and illuminated the energy cords between her and her mother.

The session culminated with radiant light. I was guided to let Barbara know that she could turn inward and pray for guidance. She didn't have to handle life's challenges alone. Again, I communicated this in the most effective way, soul to soul.

During the next few weeks, Barbara faced many difficult decisions regarding her mother's care. She prayed for help and received clear guidance at each turn. She was able to handle her mother's illness with faith and grace. Once again, her hands grew stronger.

Barbara had only those two sessions with me, but several years later, she told me that the idea that she could turn inward for help still sustained and guided her.

EMOTIONAL AND SPIRITUAL TRIGGERS FOR ILLNESS

As I have seen time and again, illness can be deeply informed by a precipitating event. Of course, Western medicine views the root cause of illness as cells gone awry or an invasion by a foreign

24

element such as a virus or bacteria. Granted, these may be the physical cause of many illnesses. But the reason we may suddenly be susceptible to a foreign invasion or find our own cells running amok may have to do with a challenge we experience in life.

The sudden death of a loved one, a broken love affair, an unfaithful spouse, or a past experience of emotional or physical abuse, can all be triggers. Yes, the dynamics in a relationship can make you sick. Healing, then, is often a question of learning new ways of behaving, thinking, and resolving emotions and beliefs.

These are just a few of the traumas that can set the stage for a physical illness. If you suddenly fall ill, you may want to think back to what happened in the weeks, months, or year or two before your symptoms began. If you can connect to the event that triggered your pain, you can get in touch with some of the root issues that might underlie your physical challenge.

You might ask yourself: *What did I feel during the traumatic event? Am I having the same feeling now, with my illness?* One woman I worked with noticed that her autoimmune disease flared up whenever her husband was especially emotionally distant and abusive. That insight eventually helped her gain the strength to leave her marriage.

For further guidance, you can also turn to Chapter 13: "Your Energy Anatomy," which explores your energy system, including the role of your chakras. Simply taking a look at the part of your body that is affected and seeing the corresponding chakra(s) may give you extra insight into your illness. For instance, if your thyroid is low functioning are you having trouble speaking up? Or, if you are having pain or illness in your heart, is there a way in which your heart has been broken? Sometimes the correspondence can be that direct.

Thinking about pain in the heart makes me think of Julia, who was diagnosed with costochondritis, an inflammation of the cartilage in the breastbone. The pain and the diagnosis came shortly after someone whom she had considered to be a friend snubbed her, as had been the dynamic of the friendship for a long time. "I would forgive her and not take her behavior personally, over and over," says Julia.

The pain and the diagnosis finally got Julia's attention, and she realized what everyone else around her knew: It was time to let go of this "friend" who was constantly breaking her heart. "I have to keep reminding myself that I have the right to pull away," she says. As Julia stepped away, she found that good things began to flow into her life. For starters, her art began to flourish.

DIFFICULT SITUATIONS

In many cases, illness forms slowly over a period of time as a person lives through a difficult situation in childhood or adulthood. He or she may not have the tools or support needed to process a difficult relationship or situation as it is unfolding, so the unresolved feelings and beliefs nest deep in the cells. I've seen many instances in which life experiences help to create physical problems. Again, the chapter on chakras may help you understand your particular situation more clearly.

The energies we repress can be very powerful, almost unbearable. I've been astonished many times by the tremendous force that can be stored in the body. Ultimately, over time, these energies can make us sick. When we add healing light these repressed energies can start to open and release.

Lee Anne, for example, had irritable bowel syndrome that was so severe that it was running her life and it was all due to repressed energies. "I just don't want to hear that there are any emotional issues," she told me when we first started working together. "I've already explored that." But the intestines and bowel, located at the second-chakra pelvic area, often relate to the ability to process emotions.

In Lee Anne's case her illness was all about unresolved emotional issues and boundary violations dating back to her childhood. A few healings helped, but she wasn't ready to deal with the childhood issues at a deeper level, and she stopped having sessions.

BLADDER PAIN: "PISSED OFF"

Some life experiences can sear so deeply that they require great fortitude and courage to overcome. Mary came to me because she had intense bladder pain. When I laid hands on Mary I ran very high frequencies of subtle energy. I quickly found that she was "pissed off"—very "pissed off." When I asked her what in her life was "pissing her off," she broke down and told me her terrible secret. Decades earlier, her husband had molested one of their young daughters, and Mary had never forgiven him.

Now that the children were grown and out of the house, she barely talked to her husband. She had banished him to the opposite end of the house. They had their own private cold war, complete with their very own Berlin Wall. But somehow, she couldn't ask him to leave—she just remained in this state of intense, cold anger.

With this teary confession, I thought, at first, that we had gotten to the root cause of her problem. But as I did a few more healings, I saw that her anger went even deeper. Yes, her husband was a worthy scapegoat, but in the end, he was just a decoy to keep the even more horrifying truth from herself and others.

The person she ultimately blamed and couldn't forgive was someone she could never escape: herself. She blamed herself for not having left the marriage and taken her daughters to safety. She confessed that when her young daughter had told her what Daddy was doing, she had pretended not to hear. Mary had been afraid that she couldn't make it as a single mother of three young children.

This was a terrible burden of guilt to carry, and I wanted very much to help Mary heal further, but she simply could not begin to forgive herself. Although she had received some relief, after a few more sessions she stopped coming.

SHOCKS TO THE SOUL

Over and over again, I have seen illness begin, intensify, or recur after a shock to the soul. One woman's multiple sclerosis was diagnosed after her husband revealed that he had been having an affair for several years and then left her. Another woman's cancer recurred when she realized that her boyfriend, with whom she had just bought a house, really wasn't a true partner, willing to be totally present and responsible. Another woman I worked with developed seizures after her beloved husband passed away from a brain tumor.

Some illnesses, particularly chronic conditions, can be the result of many different energies all coming together like a big knot. Some precipitating events are even shrouded in the mists of time. For instance, I did a healing for a woman who had lost her voice. During the session, I had a vision of her in what seemed to be an earlier incarnation. In the vision, I saw that she had silenced many people. I was shown that this was the source of her issue. She was working out that karma, or pattern, in the present lifetime.

BODY SYMBOLOGY

The aches and illnesses we get often have deep meaning; our souls express important messages to us through our bodies. For instance, I worked with a woman who called me because her breast had given off an inexplicable discharge. During the healing, I saw that her breast, a symbol of her feminine soul, was literally weeping because of an abusive dating relationship. She had just broken it off with the man in question, and as soon as she understood the deeper meaning of her physical problem, the symptom resolved.

In another situation, Cindy came to me for a healing after a melanoma was removed from her breast. I saw the underlying issue—painful experiences during her failed marriage—and cleared that energy.

She had her eyes closed during the healing. Nevertheless, on her inner mind screen she saw the energy releasing from her body. "What's that black stuff coming out of me?" she asked. I told her it was the energy from her marriage, and that now she would not have to worry about the melanoma recurring. It's been more than a decade and she has never had a recurrence.

We can learn a lot about what's going on and what we need to heal if you ask yourself: *What is my body trying to tell me? What is the symbolism?*

Take a look at the "Body Symbology" chart in Chapter 14 for some examples to help you explore. Also, in Chapter 13: "Your Energy Anatomy," you will find information about each chakra and how it relates to specific areas of the body and mind.

EVEN A CUT FINGER CAN CONVEY A MESSAGE

Remember, your soul is poetic: The message it sends to you is going to be tailored just for you. I once cut my finger, and the finger I sliced was my wedding-ring finger. At the time, I was in a relationship that everyone except me could see wouldn't lead to marriage, and this was my soul trying to draw my attention to the truth of my situation.

The message isn't always very metaphysical. Once I worked with a hostess of a holiday brunch who sliced her finger with a knife while getting all the food prepared. The message from her soul was very simple: *Slow down. Relax.* When she cut herself, she *had* to take a timeout. Brunch still unfolded beautifully, and she was amazed when a few days later, with the help of the energy I transmitted, her finger had almost completely healed.

YOUR POWER

Many illnesses involve a loss of energy. A person's energy can get knotted up due to experiences, thoughts or beliefs. When your energy is knotted, it limits access to your vitality and wisdom. By analogy, think of a garden that gets twisted, blocking the flow of water. Conversely, a person may leak energy through a lack of boundaries, self-esteem, or motivation. Again, think of a garden hose, but with holes in it. With such a hose, one can never get the full force of the water—and in the case of a person, the full force of their spirit and talents.

For instance, I've worked with numerous people who had trouble speaking up. People they loved would "walk all over them" or just do what they wanted instead of taking into consideration the wishes of their loved one. People who can't speak up will have trouble saying "No," or "Don't do that," or "That's not what I want." They can't stand in their power and express what they want or need. They leak energy by not taking care of themselves, and by suppressing anger and frustration at their situation.

Over time, though, healings can help empower them. As they receive energy, they slowly change their boundaries and gain self-esteem. They gain the power of their own voices and the confidence that they deserve to be heard, and that their wishes and needs deserve to be respected. I know all of this from the inside. Before I could heal others in this area, I had to heal my own difficulties with speaking up.

Your energy is your power: If you have lost energy, you have lost your power. Healing is often about regaining your power—learning to stand in your truth, learning to do what is right for you, learning to see others and one's self clearly. It sounds so simple, but for various reasons such simple things, things that are your birthright, may have become difficult for you to do.

ENERGY SIGNATURES

Many illnesses have an "energy signature" that is similar from one person to another. For instance, every time I've laid hands on someone with chronic fatigue syndrome, I soon feel completely exhausted. Ironically, at a deep level a person with chronic fatigue may have energy that is extremely revved up. That is what is exhausting them.

Often people who are very overweight will have a heaviness in their energy field, a density—things aren't moving. They are carrying around a lot of pain and hurt.

I can often tell if someone has high blood pressure: Typically there is a feeling of pressure in the energy field, and often there is a sense of urgency, it is quite uncomfortable, and I am not at all surprised that someone in that state might be a bit irritable or frustrated or uncomfortable. There may be underlying fear casuing some of the pressure, as well.

Meanwhile, people with anxiety almost always have a knot in their solar plexus. They aren't necessarily aware of this tension; they may have lived with it for a long time. (One man thought it was his heartbeat showing up in his abdomen.)

If you are sensitive to energy—and many people are—you will often pick up others' moods and even the energy signatures of their illnesses. You may begin to feel anxious in the presence of someone with anxiety; depressed in the presence of someone who is depressed; fearful in the presence of someone who has a lot of fear; exhausted when spending time with someone who suffers from chronic fatigue syndrome. Unless a person has had the proper training, he or she will sometimes unconsciously absorb the energies of the people with whom they spend a lot of time. This is how children absorb the energies of their parents.

If you aren't aware that you are tracking someone else's energy, you may think it's your fear, your anxiety, your sadness, your exhaustion, your anger. If you can track the feeling to its true source, that feeling will often lift from you. If you are feeling an emotional or mental state that is not normal for you, simply ask yourself: *Whose energy is this?* The answer may come to you immediately, and you will start to feel like yourself again.

YOUR SOUL'S MESSAGE IS UNIQUE

Despite these energy signatures, from an energy perspective no two people have exactly the same ailment. Your soul's message is always specific to you. Amazingly, even in two people who have the same physical issue, the underlying feeling or belief or thought will never be precisely the same.

One day some years ago, I was shown this very clearly when two people came to see me with the same problem: a pulled hamstring muscle. The hamstring is the muscle that runs up the back of the leg; you can feel it behind your knee.

Both had injured themselves in dance classes, and the injuries kept nagging at them. *What,* I wondered, *could be the big deal about a pulled hamstring muscle? Why was I getting two people with the same problem in one day?*

I soon found out. When I laid hands on the first person, Ken, who had been divorced for half a dozen years, I saw that he was feeling hamstrung. Honestly, I could not have made that one up; it was so literal that I could hardly believe it. It makes you wonder: Who made up this language, anyway?

Why was Ken hamstrung? Ken's soul showed me that he felt constricted in expressing his love. His ex-wife, Angela, with whom he was running a business, just couldn't receive these feelings from him. I helped him let go of this emotional pain, and to Ken's amazement, his hamstring muscle, which had been hurting for months, was dramatically better within a few days.

When I tuned in to the second person, Denise, an architect, I saw that she, too, felt hamstrung. In her case, the issue involved her artistic vision and creativity and her fertility. She couldn't get pregnant and hadn't worked as an architect in several years. When I connected to her energy, I was flooded with a deep existential *ennui*. I saw that whatever she did, Denise had the feeling *What's the point?* I stayed present with the feeling, bringing light to it to transform it.

Within a week of the session, Denise began working creatively again, and the transition was so natural that she didn't even associate the change in her state with the healing until a friend pointed out the synchronicity. The fertility probably would have taken a few more healings to resolve.

Both Ken and Denise were feeling hamstrung, but in completely different ways. Since that experience, whenever I do yoga, I'm always stretching my hamstring muscles to make them—and my psyche—more flexible. I don't want to be hamstrung.

Your soul's stories can be dramatic and intense, but they aren't always obvious. There are usually deep reasons why the information is stored in your body, protected from your conscious awareness. You might not have been ready to deal with the soul issue, with the intense emotions or thoughts involved, at the time it developed. The "Listening to Your Body" meditation on the next page is one way to tune in.

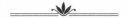

Listening to Your Body

If you have an illness, pain or discomfort, your body is trying to tell you something that's very important for you to know. If you listen it will help you heal. As you do this meditation, you may want to keep paper and a pen near you in case you want to take notes.

1. To start your meditation, turn within and focus on your breath as the breath comes in and as it goes out.

2. Allow your mind and heart to become quieter with each breath.

3. When you are very relaxed, call in the light and divine love. Also bring in your Inner Healer, the part of you that knows exactly what you need to heal.

4. When you feel very relaxed, tune in to an area of your body where you have discomfort or illness.

5. Imagine that this area is totally filled with the most radiant light.

6. Ask this part of your body: *What are you trying to tell me? What do you want me to know?* Listen carefully to whatever arises. You can jot down the impressions you receive.

7. Ask your body: *What can I do to begin to heal?* You may hear something simple—for example, that you need to rest more. Even if the answer seems obvious, listen carefully. This is your guidance.

8. When you are ready, thank the light, the part of your body that is asking for healing, and your Inner Healer. Gently come out of meditation.

9. Follow your guidance as you go about your day and your week. Your soul will communicate more and more easily with you if you respect what it tells you. (For example, it will give you more steps you can take to help you heal.)

Do this meditation as often as you like. Every time you place light into your body, it is helping you to heal. Every time you tune in to your body, you are loving and honoring yourself. Each time, you may learn something new. Notice what unfolds in your life.

THREE

Biology Is Biography

—————•••—————

YOUR SOUL'S STORY

Imagine that your body is like a book in which everything about you is recorded: your feelings, your thoughts, your beliefs, even your actions and intentions. It might read like a great autobiography if only you could decipher the code. That idea is not as farfetched as you might think—this is why one of my mentors, Rosalyn Bruyere, would often say that *biology is biography.*

As you read the cases below, allow yourself to think about your own situation and see what might begin to stir in your awareness. Having access to your true story is empowering and provides you with a key to your healing.

THE BODY TELLS THE TRUE STORY

Jason's healing story is a good example of how biology is biography. He had a healing crisis involving his eyes. The vitreous fluid in Jason's eyeball had liquefied, causing his retina to detach.

Doctors performed emergency surgery to remove the fluid and reattach the retina. "At that point," Jason recalled, "I had no idea if I would see again. I was literally in the dark. My eyeball was full of blood. There was no way of telling what the result of the operation would be. The doctors didn't know."

What could that have to do with his soul's truth? I wondered. I was working long-distance with Jason, and I told him to lie down and relax on his couch or bed while I transmitted healing light to him. When I tuned in to him, I saw that he was in a dark place metaphysically as well as literally. I could tell that he was feeling very pessimistic about his life.

This darkness was the underlying cause of his physical problem. I ran very high healing frequencies into his eye. Then I flooded his energy with the most radiant light. I showed his soul how beautiful and full of promise life could be and how wonderfully everything would turn out. By the end of the healing, I felt that the healing in his eye would unfold and that things in his life would get better.

"Fifteen or twenty minutes into the healing, I suddenly felt flooded by calm and well-being. It was absolutely tremendous," Jason recalled months later. "I had been in a very bleak place before that. Suddenly I was invaded by this lovely feeling, and I had the sense that everything was going to be all right. It was very tangible. And since then, everything has worked out very well."

Not only was Jason's eye completely healed, but also, when he went for the cataract surgery that he needed as a result of the detached retina, his vision improved more than the surgeon thought was possible. "The surgeon grins and rubs his hands when he sees me, because he's so excited," Jason says.

Most important, Jason has stepped into the light. "I didn't expect life to get so much better, but it has," he says. "Work has been coming in. And I'm back to being an optimistic person."

ECZEMA: WHO IS GETTING UNDER YOUR SKIN?

Audrey's skin had been burning and itching from eczema for about a year. "What's getting under my skin?" she wondered aloud one day to her husband. She wondered if it might be the detergent, or a new tea she had bought. "Who is getting under your skin?" he asked.

With that question, Audrey realized an acquaintance had been sucking more and more energy from her. Audrey, a natural caregiver, was giving, giving, giving. It was never enough. She stopped giving so much and the eczema improved, but only a little bit. That's when Audrey called me for a distance healing.

In the first session, I ran high frequencies into the area where she had eczema, up and down her back and along her chest. Then I strengthened Audrey's boundaries. The skin, after all, is the biggest boundary we have in our physical body. It literally encloses us. In Audrey, this boundary was distressed. I also ran energy through the cords connecting Audrey to this acquaintance with the intention for Audrey to gain the clarity she needed. When we talked at the end of the session, I helped her feel comfortable letting go of the relationship. The acquaintance was truly an energy vampire.

Audrey's eczema improved as she let go of the acquaintance, but it wasn't completely gone. In the next session, as I ran energy to clear the eczema, I saw another challenge. For years, Audrey had been home with the couple's five children. She was used to taking care of her family and their home life. But now that the last child was off at college, Audrey got swept up in traveling with her busy executive husband. Sometimes, he was going to three or four cities in a week. Flying made her anxious and the pace was dizzying. She was feeling overwhelmed and ungrounded.

For much of the session, I worked on grounding Audrey and showing her that she could stay home and tend to their home life and skip some of the trips. It would be better for both her and her husband if she took care of herself, as well as him. Plus, her husband didn't really need her on every trip either; he was busy running his business and had little time to spend with her while she was on the road with him.

After this session, Audrey's skin improved. In the third session, I continued to run energy to clear the eczema, ground Audrey, and give her the trust and understanding she needed to take time for herself. By the fourth session, Audrey was able to totally relax and be in the flow. Her skin was soon back to normal.

Simply getting in touch with the soul issue can be enough to heal a persistent problem like eczema. "It was amazing," Audrey said. "The eczema was bothering me for a year. You helped me clear it so fast. What a relief."

THE TRUTH CAN HEAL

If you want to heal a physical problem, it helps to get in touch with your deepest truth. You can often heal quite rapidly, almost miraculously so in some cases. Even after having done healings for many years, I'm still amazed sometimes to see such fast and dramatic results, often regarding problems that seemed intractable.

AN INFECTED HIP BONE

The truth not only sets us free, but also heals us, and Robert's process is another dramatic example of this principle. A high-powered media executive in his early 60s, Robert's hip-replacement surgery went awry when he developed an infection in the bone. Bone infections are insidious and dangerous, and powerful antibiotics hadn't knocked out Robert's infection.

When Robert called me for a distance healing at the urging of a friend, it was only because he was in a serious situation. He was facing a surgery in which his doctor would apply antibiotics directly to the infected bone and replace the artificial hip. If the doctors couldn't get the infection under control, he might be without a working hip for a while.

"How is your relationship with women?" I asked. I knew from the energy that this was the life issue he was wrestling with, and it was stored right in his hip, part of the area that in a Kabbalistic understanding of the body is connected to the sacredness of sexual union.

"What does that have to do with my hip?" he protested. At that moment, Robert thought I was a complete nut, and he pretty much said so. But I waited patiently. After a moment Robert decided to answer the question.

As it turned out, I had just touched on one of the most significant issues in his life. That got his attention. "Well, I've been married for more than thirty years," he told me, "but I've had my challenges in my relationships with women."

During the energy transmission, I added light to his hip to clear the infection and ran light into the relationship cords between Robert and his wife for healing, harmony, and union. A few days later, Robert told me that his wife had stayed in the hospital with him the night before surgery and they had had one of their most beautiful times together. And, he added, "I could feel tingling in the hip where you worked!" As we continued working together to heal his hip, he experienced a new connection to and love for his wife.

Although Robert started as a skeptic, we ultimately worked together for several years, first on physical healing, then on resolving anxiety, and even on various business situations as they came up.

UNEXPLAINED INFERTILITY

When Mindy came to me for a healing, she was just 28-years-old but she and her husband had been trying to get pregnant for two years without any luck. Doctors had diagnosed her with "unexplained" infertility.

As I began the healing I saw the fertility block wasn't in Mindy. Her husband, Grant, simply wasn't ready to become a father. I have seen more than a few times that a prospective father's intentions can affect whether a couple conceives. In Grant's case, I saw that his unresolved issues with his parents and fears about losing his freedom were blocking pregnancy. I began to work with Grant long distance to release his fears and then to harmonize Mindy and Grant to bring in their child. I explained what I was doing to Mindy as I worked. She was grateful for the help.

"I left your office without 'expecting' anything," Mindy told me later. "I arrived home and had a wonderful and deep sleep. The next morning I awoke feeling calmer and more accepting of my situation than I had in months. Grant and I talked. He said he did want a baby—just not with expensive doctors and high-tech procedures."

Within the month, Mindy and Grant were pregnant. "Quite a miracle and I suspect you have something to do with it," she wrote me. "It happened completely naturally, without procedures or drugs." Mindy and Grant experienced challenges as a couple, but nine months later they saw the birth of their child.

CLEARING BREAST CANCER

Miranda's case is another example of how someone can clear the underlying issues and see the illness resolve. She came for a healing session wanting to gain clarity about the best course of medical treatment for her breast cancer. She had already undergone a lumpectomy, where the tumor was removed, along with chemotherapy. But two follow-up biopsies showed she still had some stray cancer cells in her breast. Her doctors were recommending a mastectomy.

Miranda had already worked with an intuitive life coach and had cleared a number of issues before coming to me. When I laid

hands on her for the first time, I couldn't find the cancer any-
where in her breast. "I think you've cleared it," I told her.

She still didn't know how to proceed, given the medical ad-
vice she was getting. As we did healings, the same themes kept
coming up: Miranda needed to have the courage to speak her
truth and trust her intuition. She made rapid progress on both
of these issues, receiving new challenges in her life as we worked
together. She moved through her life lessons and integrated her
past quite rapidly. She was a natural at working with energy.

After a few months, her doctors pressured her again to have
the mastectomy. "I'm not sure I have cancer anymore," she said.
I agreed. I asked if she could do watchful waiting with frequent
screenings, but finally she decided that peace of mind was the
most important thing to her, as she had four young children.
She elected to have the mastectomy.

The lab report from the surgery confirmed what we both
had experienced energetically: There was no sign of cancer in
the breast that her surgeon removed. Miranda had cleared all
traces of cancer. Although Miranda technically didn't need a
mastectomy, she was happy and at peace with the result.

"It was nice to know I had really healed my issues and
cleared the cancer," she told me. "I also was glad to know that
I never had to worry about it again." She has never looked back.
She has continued to develop her intuitive gifts, and her life
has blossomed.

MISSING BLOOD PLATELETS

Sarah could process only a bit of her soul's truth at a time,
but even that little bit had a dramatic effect.

Sarah's body had pretty much stopped making platelets for
six years. There was no medical explanation and no cure. She
received transfusions every two weeks just to keep her going.
On an intuition, her chiropractor sent her to me for a healing.

After I chatted with Sarah briefly, the underlying energy cause of her platelet issue was quite obvious to me: rage. She described in vivid detail how she had felt oppressed and controlled by her mother. I could also tell that she was completely clueless about her feelings, not allowing herself conscious awareness of them even though her mother had passed away several years earlier.

If she allowed herself to see how she felt about her mother, she feared she'd lose the closeness to the one person who loved her. Her mother, at least in her mind, had always been there for her. But, in fact, her mother may have held on so tightly that Sarah never felt free to create an independent life.

Energetically speaking, Sarah's problem was actually pretty simple, although it would take time to heal. In order to suppress her rage, she had to suppress all of her "red" energy, the energy of the first chakra, responsible for vitality and healthy blood, among other things. (See Chapter 13: "Your Energy Anatomy" for more details about the first chakra.) Her body couldn't produce healthy blood cells without this energy. She would have to become aware of her true feelings to heal.

In a case like this, we go step by step. Laying hands on Sarah, I held the intention for her body to produce platelets. Almost immediately, her rage began to uncoil. Her red energy was now flowing much more freely. I knew this would have a big impact on her physical condition.

A few days after the session, Sarah's platelet levels rose dramatically for the first time since she had fallen ill. Her long-suppressed rage also rose to consciousness. In a fury, she fired every single one of her doctors.

She wasn't as upset with me as she was with her doctors. She just let me know that she was annoyed that I told her to go home and rest after the session. I'm not sure she was able to connect the rage she experienced to the session we did. But she wasn't ready to do any further healing work.

A HEALING CRISIS: IRRITABLE BOWEL SYNDROME

Harry, who had been badly abused as a child by mentally ill parents, had digestive issues for most of his life. He stored all of his feelings in his bowels and with great determination had soldiered on to become a successful functioning adult and family man. When he began to have healings, "I really want to clear this condition," he told me. "I know I'm blocking a lot of feelings. I never feel any emotions."

After just one or two sessions, Harry's anxiety went through the roof. His digestion got a little better, as the anxiety he had stored in his body came to the surface. But it was intense. The next session made things even more painful. "The spasms, nausea and anxiety are worse than ever." He told me. But Harry was determined. "I know this means I'm moving in the right direction. But it definitely is very challenging." Slowly, the enormous energy he was using to suppress his feelings will be available for a fuller and happier life. Plus, his physical discomfort will finally resolve.

As you can see from these examples, the emotional pain that we can't accept may be stored in the body, contributing to contractions in our energy and leading to illness. If you are dealing with an illness or pain, try the guided meditation, "Your Soul's Story," on the following page to get in touch with the deep meaning.

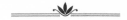

Your Soul's Story

Getting in touch with the story in your body can lead to profound healing. Here's a meditation to help you find out your deepest truth.

1. Close your eyes and watch your breath as it comes in and as it goes out.

2. Call in the light and divine love. If you wish, you may also call in your Higher Self and any healing masters or archangels to whom you feel drawn.

3. Very gently bring your awareness to a place in your body where there is discomfort or illness. Imagine that it is illuminated by radiant light.

4. Ask this part of your body: *What story are you telling?*

5. Allow yourself to be present with the story. Be the witness of it.

6. Ask this part of your body: *When did this story begin?*

7. Forgive yourself and anyone else involved in the earliest trigger.

8. Now ask yourself: *How would I like the story to be?* Can you create a version that is positive and empowering for you? This will help to change your energy and expectations.

9. See your life unfold going forward with this new story. How do things unfold. Do you make different decisions? Take different actions? Have a different perspective?

10. When you are ready, thank the light and your Higher Self or any masters or archangels you called in. Gently come out of meditation.

Do this meditation as often as you like. Many different parts to the story may emerge. Each time you create a more positive pathway, you are changing your energy and your destiny.

FOUR

Limiting Beliefs and Emotions

———— • • • ————

YOU CAN BREAK FREE

As you listen to your body and get in touch with your deepest truth, you can begin to clear stuck emotions and limiting beliefs. These stuck emotions literally cloud our understanding and responsiveness to the world. They can also help to shape our beliefs, sometimes in a way that's a distortion of the truth. In such cases, it's important to clear both the emotions and the beliefs.

BELL'S PALSY

Seemingly out of nowhere, Carl was stricken with Bell's palsy, leaving the left side of his face paralyzed. Bell's palsy can last for days, weeks or months—sometimes even years. Western medicine considers it idiopathic, meaning there is no known cause—and there is no known cure, either. But when Carl called me, I could see that there was a cause: I knew immediately that his relationship with his wife was involved.

My initial impression was soon confirmed. As I began to run energy, I saw that Carl was caught between wanting to support his wife, who was having a stressful time at work, and feeling angry about and frustrated by all the extra responsibilities that had fallen on him. These aren't uncommon feelings, of course. The difficulty was that he couldn't *face* his conflicted feelings. His emotional paralysis was manifesting in his face.

I ran many frequencies for clarity and harmony and worked on releasing Carl's anger and frustration. After the healing, Carl had an extremely vivid dream that illustrated to him exactly why he was angry. The dream also showed him where his wife was out of balance. "The dream was like no other I have ever had, and the relief was instant once I processed things," he told me.

Around that time, Carl also had a session with a practitioner of Ayurvedic medicine, the traditional medicine of India, who showed him a book that said that anger was the cause of Bell's palsy. That helped crystallize his understanding. "I was able to release a huge ball of stress that I was carrying around, and my anger was gone," says Carl. "My Bell's palsy started to fade immediately."

A few weeks later, Carl still sensed a slight weakness in his facial muscles, but no one else could detect it. He says since the healing, he's been able to recognize the stresses that upset him and then change his responses. The healing "had a significant and lasting effect. I let the anger go, and I healed. Pretty amazing!

A TUMOR IN THE EAR

Greg, a sales executive, came to me at the urging of a friend. A CAT scan had revealed an ominous shadow in his left ear. A few years earlier, a tumor had destroyed the nerve in Greg's right ear, rendering him deaf in that ear. Doctors now feared he was developing a new tumor and that he might lose his hearing altogether.

Greg didn't quite know what he was doing in a healer's office—except that he would have done anything to save his hearing. He thought his tumor was just old-fashioned bad luck. But my intuition told me there was a very real reason for his difficulties. "Did you ever have any problems with your ears before the tumor?" I asked.

"Yes," he replied. "I've been a long-distance swimmer since I was a kid. I've always had ear infections." To Greg, this was only to be expected, but I knew that not every swimmer has problems with their ears. I sensed that there was an underlying reason that Greg was having problems.

As I ran energy into Greg's ears, I immediately had a vision in which I saw him swimming in the ocean as a child, blissfully safe. The waves rocked him softly; the rays from the sun warmed him even though the water was cold; the water muffled all the other sounds of the world, creating a cocoon. I could tell that Greg was happy to be in his own world, free from the sound of other people.

I wondered, who was it that Greg didn't want to hear? The answer came in a flash: his father. Why? I asked his soul. I saw, as if watching a movie, that Greg's father had repeatedly lashed out at him.

Working energetically, I helped Greg release the anger he had built up toward his father and dissolve the belief that he needed to "turn a deaf ear." I also opened up space for him to under-stand and forgive his father. Afterward, I explained what had happened during the session. "You've just described my child-hood," he said in amazement.

At our next session a few weeks later, Greg told me he often felt intense frustration and anger at work when people didn't listen to him or, worse, raged at him. Clearly, the emotional patterns and beliefs from his childhood were shaping his life in a less than beneficial way. I helped him release the frustration and anger. I also shifted his energy so that he would be able to listen to others better. I knew that if he could listen, other people would naturally want to listen to him.

When Greg had a follow-up CAT scan, the shadow in his "good" ear was gone. His doctors gave him a clean bill of health. Moreover, Greg's healing had a particularly happy and unexpected ending: Almost two years later I ran into Greg and his wife, who casually mentioned that Greg had a 2% return of hearing in his damaged ear where the nerve had been destroyed. "The doctors couldn't believe it," she told me.

Greg's situation is not unusual. So many times when people come to me with a problem, they have emotions and limiting beliefs that are affecting their energy. When a person's emotions begin to flow and their beliefs expand, their entire life can change. Sometimes, as in Greg's case, the issues are very deep-seated. If all of the emotions and beliefs are not cleared at the root, the physical problem can recur later in life when a new stressor appears.

Creating emotional flow can be easy, and it can help you deal with any situation more effectively. Sometimes it can even diminish physical pain. Take a look at the guided meditation, "Creating Emotional Flow," to help you resolve difficult emotions.

A BELIEF THAT BLOCKED FERTILITY

Meg was only in her mid-20s but had tried getting pregnant for nearly three years without succeeding. She and her husband watched as their friends all had babies. For Meg, it was becoming difficult to celebrate everyone else's joy.

When I brought light to Meg's situation during a healing, I saw that the problem was very simple. Meg was from a very socially "proper" family. She had spent her teen and early adult years doing everything she could not to get pregnant from her relations with her boyfriend, and being mortally afraid that she might become pregnant. Her body was still carrying the old belief that pregnancy would be a disaster. I cleared that from her psyche.

I told Meg she would be pregnant in a few months. Too impatient to wait any longer, she began fertility treatment to help speed things along. She became pregnant almost immediately.

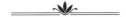

Creating Emotional Flow

As you master emotional flow, your whole life will come to a higher order. This meditation is based on Buddhist and yogic practices. It is especially beneficial if you are having a very strong emotion come up, one that almost seems to overtake you.

1. Close your eyes and watch your breath as it comes in and as it goes out.

2. When you feel very relaxed, call in the light and divine love. If you wish, you can also call in your Higher Self or a spiritual master or archangel.

3. Very gently bring your awareness to a place in your body where there is discomfort or illness. Imagine that it is illuminated by radiant light.

4. Ask this part of your body: *What feeling are you trying to express?*

5. Identify the feeling or feelings. If there is more than one feeling, choose the strongest one.

6. Allow yourself to be present with the feeling. Be the witness of it.

7. On the inhalation, breathe the feeling into your heart.

8. On the exhalation, breathe out divine love.

9. Repeat with each breath. Notice: is the feeling getting more intense?

10. If so, keep breathing in the feeling and breathing out devine love until the feeling dissipates or softens. You have just created emotional flow.

11. If you wish, bring your focus to a second and then a third strong emotion, each time repeating the process.

12. When you are ready, thank the light and your Higher Self or any masters or archangels you called in. Gently come out of meditation.

Do this meditation as often as you like. You can even do this meditation at the moment when you find yourself in a situation that creates a strong feeling, what I call an "emotional charge."

AN AMAZING REMISSION

When I saw Carol in New York, a pretty young woman in her early 30s, I thought she might have only weeks left to live. She was thin, frail, and exhausted from fighting terminal breast cancer that had invaded her bones. She was still being treated with intensive chemotherapy. She had two children who were in danger of losing their mother.

As Carol and I talked, I learned that she had recently lost both of her parents to illness; she was grieving terribly as well as facing her own diminishing life force. Soon I had her lying down and relaxing. As I transmitted healing light, I hoped to make her comfortable, but I also held the intention to heal the cancer and the underlying issue. As long as there is life, there is hope.

Soon the energy revealed something I never would have expected: Carol was being pulled toward death because she missed her parents so much. Working with her soul, I showed her that she had a choice to make: She could go to be with her parents or she could stay to mother her children.

When I left Carol, she was resting comfortably. I wasn't too confident that a single healing could pull her back into this world, but I knew I had done important work with her, clearing a belief that she needed to follow her parents.

I was as amazed as anyone—and quite thrilled—when I learned that she had gone into remission. Carol lived long enough to see her children go on to college before the cancer returned and she passed.

Perhaps you are holding beliefs that are keeping you from radiant health. Try the meditation, "Clearing Limited Beliefs," on the next page to explore and release them.

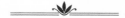

Clearing Limiting Beliefs

We all have beliefs that limit our experiences and opportunities. Sometimes these beliefs get expressed through the body. The good news is: Once you become aware of a limiting belief, you can release it.

1. Close your eyes and watch your breath as it comes in and as it goes out.

2. Allow your mind and heart to become quieter with each breath.

3. When you feel very relaxed, call in the light and divine love. If you wish, you can also call in your Higher Self or a spiritual master or archangel.

4. Very gently bring your awareness to a place in your body where there is discomfort or illness. Imagine that it is illuminated by radiant light.

5. Ask your body: *What belief are you trying to express?*

6. Now ask your body: *What is causing this belief to be there? What can I do to release it?*

7. Imagine that this belief is illuminated by radiant light. Restate it in a more positive way. For instance, let's say you find a belief that "No one cares about

me." Consciously change the thought form to, "My friends and loved ones care deeply about me and I care deeply about them."

8. When you are ready, thank the light and your Higher Self or any masters or archangels you called in. Gently come out of meditation.

9. Follow any guidance you receive.

Do this meditation as often as you like. Notice how changing your beliefs may change your ideas about what's possible and your experiences.

DRUG SIDE EFFECTS

There are many ways to find the emotions and beliefs that are weighing you down, and possibly even contributing to your illness. Side effects are one thing to explore. They can sometimes offer important, if usually overlooked, clues. In some cases, for example, the medicine a person takes for an illness will cause the symptoms to subside, but side effects such as weight gain, irritability, and depression may occur. These side effects may actually point to the energies underlying the illness. While the medicine may suppress the illness or its symptoms, the underlying emotional issues may become more obvious.

For instance, a person taking an antidepressant feels better, but the underlying emotional heaviness can express itself through weight gain. Another person may control high blood pressure with medication, but experience volatile frustration or internal pressure.

One way to work with these side effects is to first recognize they could actually be the symptoms of the deeper issues involved in your illness. Then explore these issues directly. As you work on these issues, you may also help to heal the illness. Most important, you can help to make yourself feel better emotionally.

YOUR FEELINGS ABOUT AN ILLNESS

Many people find that when they are sick or in pain different thoughts and feelings can arise. You may feel shame, anger, self-loathing, sadness, anxiety or discouragement. You may even feel you can't go on, or that life is unfair. It's a good idea to work with these feelings and release them.

As you work with these emotions that seem to be caused by your illness or injury, ask yourself: *Are these feelings and thoughts simply the result of the illness? Or did I have some of these feelings even beforehand?* The answers can be extremely valuable to you.

58

You may be surprised to find that some of these feelings and thoughts predate the illness, even if you didn't notice them earlier. For instance, an illness may cause you to feel terrible despair, but if you look more closely, perhaps that feeling of despair was there even when you were a child. Indeed, sometimes such feelings can lay the ground for the illness—or make the illness seem much worse than it might otherwise be for you.

Knowing when your difficult thoughts and feelings arose can potentially help you understand more about what is making you sick, and what you need to do to heal. The meditation, "How Does Your Pain/Illness Make You Feel?" on the next page is a good one for helping to sort these questions out.

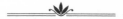

How Does Your Pain/Illness Make You Feel?

An illness or pain in the body can bring up many different thoughts and feelings. Here is a meditation to explore where and when these thoughts and feelings began—and to release what no longer serves you.

1. Close your eyes and watch your breath as it comes in and as it goes out.

2. Allow yourself to go deeper with each breath.

3. When you feel very relaxed, call in the light and divine love. If you wish, you can also call in your Higher Self or a spiritual master or archangel.

4. When you feel you are in a deep state, tune in to the area of your body where you have pain or illness. Ask your Higher Self: *What feeling or thought is my illness causing in me?*

5. Allow yourself to be present with the feeling.

6. Ask yourself: *Have I had this feeling at any other time in my life, even before my illness?*

7. Now ask yourself: *Do I need or want to keep this feeling, or can I let it go?*

8. Ask yourself: *If I was totally healed, how would I feel?* Whatever feeling comes to you—whether it's joy or peace or being centered, for instance—begin to embody that feeling now.

9. When you are ready, thank the light and your Higher Self or any masters or archangels you called in. Gently come out of meditation.

10. As you go about your day, just be present and aware of your feelings. Don't wallow in them. Don't act on them or "subscribe" to them. If you just witness the feelings, they will begin to dissolve.

11. You can add light or sweetness or acceptance whenever the feelings come up. Or do the meditation, "Creating Emotional Flow."

12. You can also begin to embody the feeling state you associate with being healed. It will help the healing integrate more quickly.

Do this meditation as often as you wish. You can continue to explore the same feeling or you can examine a different thought or feeling each time. As you explore and release difficult feelings, notice how this affects your mood, your outlook, and your experiences.

FIVE

When the Body Is Invaded

-----•••-----

WHY IS THAT INFECTION THERE?
WHAT VIBRATION IS KEEPING IT IN THE BODY?

Angela had been feeling weak for more than a year when suddenly her symptoms worsened. She couldn't walk more than a block without her legs giving out from under her. Her anxiety was spiking. She had been tested for multiple sclerosis a year earlier, but the test had come back negative. She wondered on and off if some of her symptoms might be Lyme disease. Finally she was galvanized to see a specialist. The doctor started her on antibiotics immediately, even before tests came back with a confirmation of Lyme disease.

When Angela had come for her first session a year earlier, it had been to work on her anxiety and her life. She had a good career, but in her personal life, she had retreated from new experiences and new relationships. The Lyme disease took her healing to a new level of urgency.

I felt she needed insight into what the Lyme disease might be trying to teach her. As she lay on the healing table, I invited her to journey in a guided meditation with me to the Temple of the Masters. There, flanked by three masters, we invited "Professor Lyme" to visit and talk with Angela. "What are you trying to teach me?" I instructed Angela to ask the professor.

By the end of her internal dialogue with Professor Lyme, Angela was in tears. They were tears of gratitude and understanding.

"I lost my passion for life a long time ago," she said. "Something of a despair set in. I wasn't driven anymore. I was stagnant, complacent, and fearful of moving forward. Professor Lyme attacked where I was most vulnerable."

"The disease has attacked my nervous system, mostly weakening my legs and affecting some level of my cognitive ability with loss of concentration and brain fog. The correlation: I stopped moving forward because I could not see my life clearly and all its beauty and value. The lesson? I am to appreciate and be grateful for what I have and embrace all that lies ahead. There can be no healing without an open heart and an open mind."

Angela found the guided meditation very useful: "It helped me to identify this challenge as more than just a physical ailment, but one that is also related to the emotional and spiritual. Professor Lyme embodies and keeps me focused on all three of these elements—the physical, emotional and spiritual—that need my attention, offering a triple major of study, so to speak." She said she now knew what she wanted out of life—to get better so she could live more fully.

BACTERIAL INFECTION

Our inner state can make us more—or less—attractive as a host for both bacteria and viruses. At the simplest level, we are more likely to get an infection when we are run down or under stress.

Bacterial infections may be related to a strong emotion, perhaps to an immediate but temporary situation. For example, I recently got an ear infection after I heard harsh words from someone I loved. Likewise, women sometimes get bladder infections when they are uncomfortable with something going on in their relationships but don't address it.

When powerful antibiotics are available, we don't always need to address the inner issue. Nevertheless, I recommend taking stock of the deeper meaning of an infection in conjunction with taking any needed antibiotics. This way you will bring your life to a higher order and fully recover. You will also be less likely to get sick again.

With so many bacteria becoming resistant to antibiotics nowadays, we may be called upon increasingly to look at the inner issues. Hospitals have become particularly dangerous places where drug-resistant diseases sometimes flare up. We often forget how virulent bacterial infections can be, but I have seen firsthand that they are no joke.

VIRAL INFECTIONS

Viruses are another story. They are often an invitation to change deep patterns, beliefs, and behaviors. (In some ways, chronic Lyme disease functions more like a virus than a bacterium.)

If you have a chronic virus like Epstein-Barr, ask yourself: *What is exhausting me?* There may be many factors at play when you have a chronic viral condition. Did you push yourself beyond your limits before falling ill? Why? You may have experienced emotional abuse in your childhood of which you are unaware, or merely an extreme pressure to perform and be perfect. Often there is a call to strengthen your boundaries and stand up for yourself and nurture yourself.

Even if someone tells you your chronic mystery illness is the result of a virus, the deeper questions remain: Why is your system hosting this virus? How can you release it? Finding the answers to these questions will help you heal all aspects of your life.

Try the guided meditation, "Meeting With the Spirit Form of Your Illness," at the end of this chapter to explore these questions.

A CASE OF HERPES

Many years ago a young actress, Louise, came to me for a healing. Her boyfriend had given her herpes. Afterward, he claimed that he hadn't known he had the infection. By the time Louise came for help, she was in a terrible state, having had a painful, nonstop herpes outbreak for months, pretty much since the initial infection.

As she told her story, it was clear that she was very upset with her boyfriend but wouldn't allow herself to know it. Instead she was clinging to him, afraid that no one else would ever want to be with her. Meanwhile, he was planning to move to a new city—without her.

As I laid hands on Louise, I saw that the virus was very attracted to her agitation and distress, just the way a child will be drawn to candy, or a cat to a sunny, cozy place to nap. I also saw that her agitation and distress wasn't new. Her father had constantly disregarded her boundaries. This issue is what made her so "tasty" to the herpes virus.

The virus was functioning in the same way as her father's energy. Because of that, she had no boundary that would keep it at bay. When I told her what I had seen regarding her father, she knew exactly what I was talking about, although she had never noticed it or had words for it before.

Louise needed better boundaries, and I held energy for her to stand up for herself. I also released a great deal of the agitation in her energy field. Soul to soul, I showed her that she deserved to be loved and cherished and respected and that she didn't need this boyfriend, who had not treated her well.

It was six months before I heard from Louise again. She said she had left my office knowing that her infection would get worse before it got better, and indeed it had, as can happen in a classic healing crisis event. Then it had cleared. She had been free of any recurrence since then. Just bringing it to consciousness, had been enough to release her from the virus's grip.

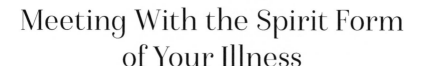

Meeting With the Spirit Form of Your Illness

Every bacterium and virus has a spirit form. You can meet with your illness to see how it wants to help you heal. On the surface the illness may seem like anything but a friend. But on a deeper level it may be helping your spiritual and personal growth in profound ways. You may want to do this meditation even if you are taking medicine for an infection. It may help you heal faster or more completely.

1. Close your eyes and witness your breath as it comes in and as it goes out. If your breath is rapid or uneven, don't worry. Just watch it come in and go out. It will eventually become more even and deeper.

2. Allow your mind and heart to become quieter with each breath.

3. When you feel very relaxed, imagine you are vising a beautiful Temple of Healing, where everything is radiant with spiritual light.

4. Let your Higher Self or a healing master come to meet you and bring you into a special room for healing. Whatever you imagine or see in your mind's eye is perfect.

5. Invite the spirit form of your illness to come meet with you. What does he/she/it look like or feel like?

Even a fleeting impression is useful. It's OK if you think you are making it up—just go with what comes to you.

6. Ask the illness why it has come and what you can learn from it.

7. Listen carefully to the answer, even if you think you are making it up. You can dialogue with the spirit form of the illness.

8. Thank the illness for being a teacher and thank your Higher Self and any master who has been with you. Gently come out of meditation.

Work with the wisdom and strength the illness is giving you. See how you can incorporate these gifts as you go about your day and your week.

SIX

The Healing Process

∙●∙

INNER AWARENESS OPENS SLOWLY, LIKE THE PETALS OF A LOTUS BLOSSOM

People often ask me, "How long will it take to heal?" The answer: "How deep a transformation do you want?" Healing is a little like a cleaning project. Let's say you clean a shelf in your kitchen cabinet. When it's orderly and sparkling, you realize you could clean all the other shelves in the cabinet. In fact, you could clean *all* of the shelves in *all* of the cabinets. Likewise, when you heal one thing, sometimes that's enough, and at other times you realize you want more order and sparkle everywhere.

Over time, I've healed many different things in myself. Each time I heal a pattern I go on to a deeper level and to new issues. I do this because it enhances my life so much. Healing one thing often leads to healing another. As you work with one layer, you discover what's beneath it and you may want to heal that, as well.

As you heal, you will feel lighter and happier; your symptoms will soften or disappear. I've seen cancer markers dissolve. Perhaps even more powerful, I've witnessed deep transformations in people's lives, such as the resolution of long-standing emotional and physical challenges and limiting beliefs.

Occasionally, there is an immediate and dramatic healing of a chronic issue. Usually, however, transformation takes time. I've seen people give up after just one or two healings because they didn't see a powerful result. Whatever healing process you are using, give it some time.

Conversely, you can often see dramatic results. Indeed, sometimes the healing process can even cause a brief intensification of the very symptoms you are healing. It usually lasts just a few days. It is auspicious, although not easy to tolerate. Among healers, this effect is called a healing crisis. It is, alas, very common. As some of the energy causing your problem leaves the body, you can have a heightened awareness or experience of it.

Over time the incremental changes begin to add up. One day you realize you're a new person, living in a new way.

A CASE OF ARRHYTHMIA

Healing is like reshaping a geological landscape. It can be hard work and take a lot of energy. It can be a process rather than one "miraculous" event.

This was the case for Jim, a business coach who had a persistent and relatively intense arrhythmia. He was having frequent episodes in which his heart would suddenly start to beat wildly out of control. His heart would go into these spasms even though he was taking medicine to prevent such incidents. It was unnerving and frightening. Afterward, he would feel shaken.

Jim never knew when an episode would happen—he could be in a restaurant, in his office, or walking down the street. I happened to witness one of these events so I could see how scary it was. I ran energy until the episode resolved. After that, Jim decided he would work on the underlying energy of his arrhythmia, and he came to me for support.

As I laid hands on Jim, I could feel a distinct tightness in his heart that echoed painfully in my own heart. Soon I heard the title of Maya Angelou's famous autobiography, *I Know Why the*

Caged Bird Sings. Then I knew: Jim's soul wanted to be free of the constriction in his heart.

Jim didn't know there was a constriction in his heart; that was the way things had always been. He could point to a repressive atmosphere in his childhood, but the emotional and spiritual constriction had stayed with him through his adulthood without his conscious awareness. Now his soul was like a caged bird flapping its wings wildly to be free. This was the cause of his episodes of arrhythmia.

I worked with Jim's energy to loosen the tightness in his chest. I also transmitted frequencies for joy, harmony, clarity, and flow to help give his heart a more fluid pattern. When the session ended, Jim felt very relaxed, but I could see that he was thinking, *Is that it?*

The effects of energy aren't always immediate. They seep in slowly and organically. Sometimes the changes seem so natural that people don't even notice they've had a shift. Being in balance simply feels right.

Jim and I did about half a dozen sessions over three months. Each time, I focused on expanding and freeing his heart rhythm. We explored his childhood and his present life and the places where he felt stuck. We also examined the relationships in his life in which he wished for more connection. Jim looked forward to our sessions and enjoyed them. His arrhythmia eased a bit, but it wasn't completely gone.

Jim soon got busy with other things and stopped coming for sessions with me. However, not long after our sessions ended, he began taking a more spiritual approach in his business coaching. He was excited by the breakthrough and pleased that clients appreciated this new openness. Jim did not associate this shift with the healings, but I did. As he opened his heart, his arrhythmia faded away.

"The arrhythmia is definitely better," Jim told me when I checked in with him 18 months after our last session. "I went through a period where it was minimal. I would have an occasional flutter maybe every few weeks for an hour. It was really minimal." He even lowered his medicine to half the prescribed dose.

Right around the time I checked in, the arrhythmia had "popped up" again. His doctor had put him back on a full dose of medication. I interpreted this resurgence to mean that his soul wanted even more opening in the heart. But Jim was just happy that for now, at least, his medicine actually worked.

More than five years later, when I checked in again, Jim told me that over the course of four years he had had two surgical procedures called ablations to neutralize the area producing the arrhythmia. Finally, a pacemaker combined with daily meds had solved the problem. He believes that he, like everyone else, only accepts data that supports his beliefs. "There probably wasn't room in my 'bubble' to allow your healing to take," he says. I might agree—I always had the feeling that if Jim had continued with the healings, it would have helped physically, emotionally, and spiritually.

ECZEMA: PEELING THE LAYERS

In healing deep patterns there can be ups and downs, remissions and intensifications. It's a journey. Over time the original pattern becomes a faint shadow or completely dissolves.

Amy's case is another example of how a "simple" physical problem can open doors in a person's life. She called me for help with a terrible bout of eczema on her hands. They were inflamed and itching. Indeed, the burning was so terrible that she often scratched her skin until it was raw. Overall, she was feeling miserable.

Amy's eczema was a bit more complex than Audrey's, which I discussed in Chapter 3. The frustration Amy was experiencing was much deeper and she had been suffering from eczema longer and more intensely. Amy's husband had lost his job a few years back; over time they had run out of money. Interestingly, the inflammation in her hands had begun shortly after her husband lost his job. But she hadn't linked these two things until her session with me.

When Amy contacted me, her husband was finally working again, but they were buried in debt from the two years he had been unemployed. His financial problems had gotten under her skin in a big way. It was almost more than she could handle. As I ran energy into Amy's hands, I saw that she had a lot of pent-up anger and resentment toward her husband. I helped release some of the frustration and anger. I also worked on empowering Amy.

In the next healing more details emerged. Amy felt that her husband was not responsible enough around money. Plus, she was still bitterly angry at how he had handled things during his unemployment. I worked on releasing these feelings, and putting light on bringing her life to a higher order and strengthening her boundaries and resolve.

After just a few sessions, Amy began to turn things around. She got part-time work. She sat down with her husband and went over their financial information. She took over paying all their bills. She and her husband also worked on their communication to improve their marriage. Her eczema had dramatically improved. The full healing would take time, but Amy was on her way.

TWISTS AND TURNS: SCOLIOSIS

Healing isn't always as straightforward as we might like it to be. We can't know exactly what the path will look like until it unfolds. When we add light we can trust that the process is always moving a person to a higher order. But sometimes it can seem as they've temporarily taken a turn for the worse. Healing follows its own mysterious course.

Matt had been diagnosed with scoliosis, a curvature of the spine, when he was just a little more than 3-years-old. Rods were placed in his back, along his spine. Although they didn't actually straighten the spine, they gave his organs the space to grow normally. By the time Matt's parents brought him to see me, he was 10-years-old and had been having surgeries almost every nine months for most of his life. He suffered through them gallantly. Nevertheless, they took a toll on him and his family.

My first goal was to give Matt comfort before, during, and after his surgeries. I also worked on alleviating the trauma that was already in his body. At the same time, I always held the intention for Matt's spine to straighten. The surgeries got easier for Matt to handle. But after several surgeries I began to sense that his body did not welcome the rods. When I mentioned this to his parents, I was told that the rods were critical in helping Matt grow in a healthy way.

About two months after a routine surgery, Matt had a severe physical reaction to the rods. The rods were quickly removed, along with the hardware that held them in place. Afterwards, I did several long distance healings focused exclusively on straightening Matt's spine. I could literally feel his spine straighten as I worked. Of course, I didn't know what that would look like in the physical domain. But it was such a powerful feeling that I believed something would manifest on the physical plane. Nevertheless, such an occurrence would be so dramatic that I couldn't assume something physical would happen.

When Matt had his first set of scans following the rod removal, the pictures showed that his spine had straightened by nearly 20 degrees. I was amazed and delighted. His surgeon thought he was looking at the wrong set of scans. Even after he double-checked, "he wouldn't believe the radiologist's report," Matt's father told me. "He had to measure the angles himself. He had never seen this kind of improvement." Matt's father said that when the doctor accepted that the result was real, he was "grinning ear-to-ear with happiness."

It was a transformation for Matt's father, too. "My faith in and knowledge of the efficacy of light energy is fully committed now," he told me.

As Matt's case demonstrates, there can be many twists and turns in healings. Indeed, despite this miraculous straightening, there were more challenges for Matt, including a collapse of the spinal bones behind his heart. At that point, he received one final surgery to insert a permanent rod that would keep his spine straight in adulthood. I have learned to trust that all of what occurs is designed to bring everything in our lives to a higher order.

A HEALING CRISIS

When there is an intense issue in the body, the healing process can often involve a healing crisis. As the energy causing the illness gets released, it can cause a brief intensification of the physical challenge or the underlying emotional issue that could last from a few days to a week. For instance, ringing in the ears can intensify before it releases; anxiety can get more extreme before peace settles in; pain can briefly become worse before it resolves.

In some cases, the healing process involves a series of healing crises. I experienced this as I healed my migraines and anxiety. There would be flare-ups every time I had a healing. This went on for a very long period of time. But eventually these energies resolved.

A good analogy is: It's when you take out the garbage, that you notice the smell the most. Or when you first open a bottle of perfume, the fragrance is most intense.

These healing crises can be arduous to endure. They show you just what is really being stored in the body. It can take a lot of fortitude, and even courage, to persevere.

MULTIPLE ISSUES

People often have several different problems, all seemingly unrelated. However, quite often everything fits together when viewed at a deeper level. I worked with a man who developed rheumatoid arthritis sometime after surgery corrected his Crohn's disease. The same energy conditions were at the root of both conditions. In other cases, a person may have a physical problem and not connect it to an emotional challenge. For instance, a flare-up of herpes may occur after stress in a relationship.

Rose's situation is a perfect example of this phenomenon. She had just signed divorce papers when she called me to regain emotional stability. Her husband had filed for divorce against her wishes, after having had an affair. "By the way," she added, "I also have hemorrhoids. Is there anything you can do about that?"

We were working at a distance. As I laid my energy hands on Rose, I saw almost immediately that Rose felt that her husband had been mean to her. As a rule, I don't use rough language, but Rose's soul wasn't about to mince words. I heard that "her husband had been an ass—." I saw that she was definitely going to be better off without him. I also saw that this was something she had never admitted to herself.

"My God," Rose said, excitedly when I explained what I had seen. "I did feel my husband was "an ass—!" But I never would have said that. I loved him. But you know, it's funny—I did notice that my hemorrhoids would act up when I was upset with him."

A month later, Rose called. "Can there be a delayed reaction to a healing?" she inquired. "Because a little while after the healing, my hemorrhoids completely disappeared. I had had them for years. Thank you so much."

Sometimes bringing radiant light to the body or situation in your life can help resolve it. You can try working with the guided meditation, "The Light of Awareness," on the next page to bring a deeper understanding.

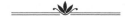

The Light of Awareness

When you place light into your body or a problem in your life, it will bring you new understanding. You may think you are imagining the light. But it is real. And it is very healing.

1. Gently close your eyes and tune in to your breath as it comes in and as it goes out.

2. When you feel very relaxed, call in the light and divine love. If you wish, you can also call in your Higher Self.

3. Think about one difficulty—physical, emotional or experiential—you have been trying to heal, perhaps for a very long time.

4. Hold this issue in the light of awareness. Make your mind very radiant. Let the issue be illuminated as it rests in this radiance.

5. When you are ready, thank the light and your Higher Self. Gently come out of meditation.

Do this meditation as often as you like. Notice what unfolds. Be detached from results. Whenever we hold an expectation, it can interfere with the free flow of energy.

REPROGRAMMING THE UNIVERSAL FIELD

We all live in an infinite universe of energy. Your individual energy field is connected to this universal field. So when you shift, it affects this universal field, not just your body and your emotions. (This is why techniques to manifest your desires and dreams work.)

As you shift, the circumstances of your life shift. Thus, working with healing energy, including prayer, can bring about creative solutions to problems. The universe will even send the right help.

Hilda's situation is an example. A bunion on her right foot became infected and turned gangrenous, and the doctors wanted to amputate part of her foot. At the request of her daughter, I did a healing for Hilda. I saw that her body had stored her anger at her ex-husband in that toe joint. Even though they had divorced decades earlier, that anger was still there.

I helped to release the anger that was causing the inflammation. I was confident that Hilda's toe would heal now, but it didn't get much better in the next day or two. Doctors were preparing to do the amputation. I just didn't see that being necessary, based on the energy and, fortunately for Hilda, my perception turned out to be right. A new doctor arrived on the scene and he came up with an innovative treatment protocol involving a hyperbaric chamber. It saved Hilda's foot.

Leslie is another example of someone who was sent the exact physical help she needed to solve her problem after her healing. She was having fainting spells, and her regular doctor had diagnosed her as being iron-deficient. But even with transfusions, she wasn't getting better. In fact, her blood pressure was dangerously low. Leslie began to have dreams that she would die. During a long-distance session I saw that everything was going to be fine.

"It's something very minor," I told Leslie. "Something to do with the salts or minerals in your body being out of balance. It's going to be very easy to fix." I held light for her to find the right doctor who could give her the proper supplement. A day later, a Chinese herbalist told Leslie that she had a calcium deficiency and gave her an herbal remedy. Soon, she was back to normal.

DEEP TRANSFORMATION

Some of the most intense healings I have witnessed and helped to facilitate involve people facing a terminal illness. As I mention in various places in this book, I have seen people recover from stage III and stage IV cancer. But some of the deepest transformations I have seen have been in people who ultimately passed on. Everyone here on this planet is destined to pass. But we can do so in an illuminated way. The soul continues on. The body is a vehicle that has served its purpose. That is what dies when the soul leaves.

Many years ago I worked with Claire, a woman in her late 60s who had been diagnosed with leukemia, on healing her body. She lived several years longer than her doctors had predicted— and always with vitality, able to enjoy her grandchildren, walks in nature, and time with her husband.

The most remarkable part of Claire's healing was that she discovered that she had a soul. Our long-distance sessions, in which she could feel me from hundreds or thousands of miles away, gave her the understanding that she was not her body. She became metaphysical in other ways as well. As she lived with her "terminal" diagnosis, she would read in the newspapers about people who passed from natural disasters and accidents.

Her sense of the mystery and wonder of life grew with each day, along with her gratitude and amazement. Claire deeply touched friends and family with a regular letter she wrote in which she shared her subtle perceptions and her gratitude for the beauty of life. She passed in an elevated state.

Phillip, too, had a transcendent experience as he faced lung cancer. At first he was focused on healing his illness. One day, I asked him what he would like to do, if and when he recovered. At that moment, Phillip realized that there was nothing left that he needed or wanted to accomplish. This was transformative. He quickly accepted that he would be passing. From then on, he was at peace with his situation and his life.

In the following weeks and months, he came to realize his many metaphysical gifts and all the goodness and love he had brought to the people in his life. His understanding of his greatness and his spiritual gifts of love, compassion and insight to others blossomed. He let go of all the anger and sadness that had entangled him for many years.

Phillip spent his last months loving all of his friends and his family, and listening with his heart. I still think of him and experience his presence. When Phillip died, his wife told me it was a sacred experience, much like when she gave birth.

All healings involve the soul. But sometimes a healing is simply for the soul, and these are truly among the most powerful healings of all.

SEVEN

Chronic Conditions

———— • • • ————

A BIG KNOT IS OFTEN MADE UP OF
MANY SMALLER KNOTS

C hronic illness is painful, discouraging, and limiting. If you've been sick or in pain for a while, healing will most likely take some time. The good news: healing energy can immediately begin to release the knots that led to the chronic condition. You can start to feel better instead of worse with each passing week, month and year.

The subtle energy used in healing and the guided meditations in this book can give you hope, relief, and comfort—and help you begin to resolve the underlying issues making you sick. When we talk about "subtle" energy, some people may think the energy is insignificant. But this energy is both fundamental and extremely powerful. As one person who received a few healings on my table said, "It didn't feel like much had happened during the session. I just felt a little drowsy. But the effect the healing had was incredible, resulting in a resolution of my symptoms and a life-changing transformation."

When you have a chronic illness, it is an opportunity for radical self-discovery, whether you were looking for it or not. Truly, you are not alone. In our culture, chronic illness is epidemic. The Centers for Disease Control and Prevention estimates half of all adults in the United States have some form of chronic illness, whether it is diabetes, heart disease, alcoholism, obesity, irritable bowel syndrome, cancer, or any number of other conditions. Western medicine can manage many of these illnesses, but often offers little in the way of healing.

When there is a chronic illness or condition, you may have many different emotions, thoughts, beliefs and behavioral patterns that feed into it. Even when you gain clarity about any one of these patterns, it can continue to recur from different angles or levels of subtlety. Thus, a chronic condition may present you with the journey of a lifetime.

As you focus on healing you may see progress immediately, or you may feel you released one knot after another but find the chronic condition hasn't budged—yet. Either way, it is a deep process. Take heart. If you work with the energies you will go in the right direction.

What is ultimately healed will be much more than your physical challenge. For instance your gastrointestinal difficulties may be a call from your soul to heal your lack of boundaries, so that people can no longer take advantage of you. Or perhaps you are being asked to digest emotional information more effectively. The physical illness generally will heal along with the underlying issues.

If you are chronically overweight, you will most likely be able to shed pounds—and keep them off—as you become aware of the emotional patterns and pain weighing you down. Maybe someone in your childhood didn't treat you right. Or maybe someone violated your boundaries emotionally or physically or sexually. Or perhaps someone gave you candy rather than emotional support.

As you become aware, you can release these underlying patterns and emotions. If you do your inner work, you can truly free yourself of the lingering effects of your past and live a much freer and more fulfilling life. The healing can be on all levels when you work with the subtle energies.

To help you in your healing process, you can use any or all of the guided meditations in this book. The important thing is not to get discouraged. Everyone wants to be healed instantly. As a healer, I always wish I could wave my magic wand and give instant healing, but a chronic condition usually requires patience and fortitude. Know that as you heal, you can create dramatic transformation. Use the guided meditation, "Seeing Progress," on page 85 to become aware of how much you've accomplished already.

One thing to keep in mind is that flare-ups of a chronic condition are often a form of guidance. Your soul is trying to get your attention. When you begin to understand your emotional and spiritual triggers, you can see what your body and soul are trying to tell you. Thus your illness is, in a strange way, actually your friend and spiritual guide.

MIGRAINE HEADACHES

I will use myself as an example here. For most of my life I suffered from migraine headaches, but except during the times I was having one, I never gave it a second thought. It was only when I began to investigate healing that I realized I had a chronic condition. When I look back, my lack of insight into my situation boggles my mind, but that was where I was at that time.

It took me years of working with these headaches to figure out what triggered them. The first level involved obvious things like getting enough rest and food when my body needed it. Eventually I got down to much deeper levels. I realized my headaches sometimes occurred when someone I cared about wasn't as loving or present as I wanted or expected him or her to be.

Because I subconsciously couldn't let myself see this, I would contract my energy and get a headache. (You could say that my migraines were about "blinding pain.") Another trigger was feeling obligated to do something that was not in my best interest, forcing myself to proceed even though on a subconscious level I knew it wasn't the right action for me.

Once I recognized my major triggers, I was able to prevent some headaches simply by seeing a situation clearly and listening to what my guidance told me to do. When I did get a headache, I knew my body was trying to tell me something. My headaches were debilitating, but now I understood that they were actually a form of guidance: My soul was speaking to me—loudly. Not even migraine medicine would help until I allowed myself to see what was really going on, at which point my headache would lift.

Even after I figured out these triggers, I had yet another layer to heal. At a primal level, my headaches were a reaction to fear. Many of us have deep levels of fear, whether we are aware of it or not. Indeed, fear is so deep in so many of us that the Indian masters and gods are often depicted with their hands in the Indian *mudra* (position) for fearlessness.

This fear was embedded deep in the core of my energy. It could be triggered by a new event or by having to step forward in new ways. I had to slowly unravel it in my head, third eye and my gut. Eventually, I was able to access the vibration of fear when it arose from my core and begin releasing it from my field.

It took me years to heal these layers and there's still more to do. But I thank God every day that I have released so much. The healing process has empowered me on many different levels, as well as freeing me from moments of intense physical suffering.

My migraines have already given me so many gifts. Without them I might not have become such a focused meditator—or such a powerful healer. Whenever I'm not well I meditate until I get better. Over time I have been able to access very subtle levels of my being. My headaches also led me to change my interactions with myself and others. Ultimately, my headaches also led me to heal my vision on all levels, as I discuss in the next chapter.

In order to heal, you have to be ready to see more clearly. Then you can take active steps to live in alignment with your soul's wishes. To explore the gifts your illness has given you, try the guided meditation, "Finding The Silver Lining," at the end of this chapter.

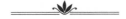

Seeing Progress

If you have been on a healing journey, it is important to acknowledge the progress you are making—even if you haven't reached your goal.

1. Gently close your eyes and tune in to your breath as it comes in and as it goes out.

2. When you feel very relaxed, call in the light and divine love. If you wish, you can also call in your Higher Self or a spiritual master or archangel.

3. Bring into your awareness an issue you have been trying to heal, perhaps for a very long time.

4. Think of one way in which you have made progress. If more than one example comes into focus, acknowledge each event.

5. Now think about why you want to heal this pattern. Ask yourself: *How will my life be different when this is finally healed?*

6. Think of one thing you can do to shift your life toward achieving this goal.

7. Now ask yourself: *How will I feel when I'm healed?* Perhaps you'll feel confident, or be at peace, or be joyful.

8. Begin to embody whatever feelings you associate with being healed.

9. When you are ready, thank the light and your Higher Self or any masters or archangels you called in. Gently come out of meditation.

As you go about your life, start making the changes that you've been shown will help you move forward. Also continue to embody the feeling you associate with being healed. Notice what unfolds.

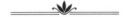

Finding the Silver Lining

It can seem as if there is nothing redeeming about your illness. But it can help you heal if you can find the good things that have come to you. You may even be surprised to see there is goodness.

1. Gently close your eyes and tune in to your breath as it comes in and as it goes out.

2. When you are in a deep space, call in the light and divine love.

3. Bring into your awareness an issue that you have been trying to heal, perhaps for a very long time.

4. Think of one way in which this very painful problem may have a silver lining. For instance, pain might force you to retreat and take much-needed time for yourself, or it might bring you the attention you need from a friend or loved one.

5. Thank the illness for giving you this gift.

6. Ask yourself: *Can I give myself this gift, even without the illness?* Set your intention to give this gift to yourself.

7. Now ask your Higher Self to show you another gift you have received from this illness.

8. Again, look at how you could give yourself this gift, even if you weren't ill. Set your intention to give this gift to yourself.

9. When you are ready, thank the light and gently come out of meditation.

As you go about your life, begin to freely give yourself the gifts you relied on your illness to give you. Also thank your illness each time you receive one of these silver linings. Notice what unfolds.

EIGHT

Genetic or Energetic?

—— •●• ——

WE INHERIT ENERGIES AS WELL AS GENES

M any people have what seem to be genetic issues. A physical challenge is passed down through the genera- tions. Sometimes it can be seen in various branches of the family tree: in aunts, uncles, or cousins as well as parents, siblings, and children. Nevertheless, what seems to be completely genetic can have energetic components. Even if you have a fam- ily history of heart disease, for example, that doesn't mean all is dictated by genetics. Some of the heart disease running through your family history could be due to a family history of energy patterns, such as a tendency towards anger, suppressed emotions, or being extremely driven.

We learn these family energy patterns even before we can talk; they are transmitted as effectively as genes. Indeed, as each of us gestates in our mother, we are resting in her womb, right at her second chakra. Because that is the center that processes emo- tion, we are literally marinating in our mother's emotional body. (See Chapter 13: "Your Energy Anatomy.") We are deeply affected by our mother's thoughts and beliefs. Everything in her energy field feeds our energy.

The heart creates the biggest electromagnetic frequency in the entire body, permeating every cell. During gestation we feel the unique rhythm of our mother's heart. If our mother is anxious, we will feel that. If she is depressed, we will experience that. If she is happy or sad, we get those vibrations, too. After we are born, we continue to be bathed in the energies of our parents and other close relatives as we grow up.

I'm not saying genes don't play a part in your physical make-up or your physical problems, just that it may not all be in your genes, whether you are dealing with bunions or heart disease or nearsightedness. Even in the scientific community, there's growing consensus (mainly based on identical-twin studies) that how you live your life is just as important as your genes.

This is good news. It means that some disease patterns can be alleviated through energy healing. This doesn't apply, of course, to diseases such as Huntington's disease and conditions such as Down syndrome, for which there are clear genetic markers. However, even when a genetic disorder exists, it seems that stress and other factors can act to intensify or alleviate the problem. In some genetic conditions, there is a range of expression of genes. In those situations, sometimes just being more peaceful can alleviate the intensity of the gene expression.

By all means do everything your medical doctors recommend. But don't give up on healing yourself on the emotional, mental and energetic levels—you might be surprised by how much your physical situation can improve. At the very least, you will be in a higher emotional flow and enjoy life more.

NEARSIGHTEDNESS: A PERSONAL EXAMPLE

I have been nearsighted since third grade. I can thread a needle by looking at it closely, but I need glasses to see most of the world around me. I couldn't even see my way around my kitchen without glasses. For many years, I assumed the problem was genetic. When I was a child, my mother was very nearsighted, and my dad was moderately nearsighted. Everyone assumed that I had inherited those genes.

But in 2006, right around when Independence Day is celebrated in the United States, I decided to put my understanding of healing to the test. Could I heal my eyes—and by doing so, could I heal some deep underlying issues, ones I perhaps didn't even know that I had?

I started this healing process by doing some Bates method exercises (a system for naturally improving eyesight) to loosen the fixed rigidity of my eyes. When I started my experiment, I was so nearsighted that I couldn't read a book without glasses; I'd have to hold it so close to my face, I couldn't see a whole page. Even so, the Bates method instructor I consulted told me I would have to stop using my full strength eyeglass prescription in order to give my eyes the room to heal. With the Bates method, the idea is that the "crutch"—the full-strength glasses—must be removed so the eyes can begin to work again.

I was practically in tears the first few nights. Even with contact lenses at half the strength of my regular prescription, I could barely see anything. I could not even function in my own kitchen; everything was a blur.

I spent the first year walking along the beach every afternoon, using a shifter (a broad piece of board with lots of thin slats) across my eyes as I walked. The shifter was designed to disturb the fixed position of my nearsighted eyes. Slowly, I began to see details that I hadn't known existed. I found that I could make out a thin stretch of telephone wires. Watching these wires became one of the signature ways in which I measured my progress.

I also had many healing sessions with one of my mentors, Rosalyn Bruyere, a phenomenal healer whom many consider "the godmother" of modern healing because she has influenced so many healers. Rosalyn helped release an enormous amount of tension around my eyes and in my entire head. She also helped me to contemplate the many things I couldn't see about myself and my family and the world around me. There were many emotional levels to clear. The confusion and frustration of not being able to see was there at the beginning. Later, a lot of anger and frustration came up, all of it stored in my eyes. Eventually that cleared, and beneath it I found a deep layer of sadness. I also began to see different aspects of my childhood, my relationships, and the arc of my life.

As I began to see more clearly on emotional and spiritual levels, my vision continued to improve. I ultimately went from glimpsing one little stretch of telephone wires—in a "now you see it, now you don't" sort of way—to seeing the wires stretching out all the way into the distance.

Now, a decade after starting the process, I can read street signs without glasses when I drive during the day. When I go to the beach, I can see the faces of people around me. I can swim and lift my head out of the pool and see my husband or my son standing at the far side of the pool. I can even read a book now without needing glasses. For me, these things are a miracle.

I've basically gone from being someone who was essentially completely visually handicapped without glasses to being someone who can see—but I still don't have 20/20 vision. Even during the day there is some blurriness, especially at long distances. And I don't see very well at night, or indoors, or in poor lighting; I still rely on my glasses in those circumstances.

The Bates instructor told me that my eyes would still adjust to as much prescription as I used to wear. But in my case, although I can see perfectly with my old prescription, it feels too strong for my eyes and causes them to hurt. Despite the fact that I haven't reached 20/20 vision, I've had a miraculous healing, and my vision continues to improve in its incremental way. I don't know where the endpoint will be.

During the time of healing my vision, I have fulfilled many personal wishes that had been out of my reach, including getting married and having a child. These may seem like simple things to most people, but to me they were major healings. Obstacles that had been in my way were lifted. I share this experiment and its amazing results because it is proof of something I've long contemplated: Many of the things that we think are genetic are actually energetic.

In the healing community, there is a theory that to heal a pattern takes as long as the pattern has existed. That would mean that as far as my vision goes, I have about 30 more years of healing to go. I don't exactly subscribe to that theory. But healing a deep pattern can require patience. I am thrilled with the progress I've made, and anything more will be icing on the cake.

BUNIONS

In addition to healing my eyesight, I also tackled the bunions I've had on both feet since my early twenties. I had always assumed my bunions were genetic and would only get worse. My maternal grandmother had such terrible bunions that she had to cut open her shoes. My father also has serious and painful bunions, as does one of my maternal first cousins.

My bunions were painful, and so bad that the joints were frozen. But through a combination of gentle yoga and occasional energy work I have done for myself, I have opened up the joints in both of my feet over the past fifteen years. I released some intense emotions that were stored in the joints as I did this work. When I experienced pain and stiffness in the bunions, I got in touch with feelings of frustration and anger. I dissolved these feelings, and the stiffness in the joints, at the same time.

Now I have much more mobility than I did when I started years ago, and one foot is so open that the pain has disappeared. The bone in that joint still juts out, but there is no bulge or swelling in the joint. The other joint is still opening and still feels slightly painful sometimes.

EXPLORING THE ENERGIES

Even if you have a health challenge in which genetics are a factor, you can still explore the emotional and energetic components and heal on those levels. That alone can be profound. And, it is possible, in some cases, it can ameliorate the physical effects as well. You can start by asking yourself: *When did I start getting symptoms? What was going on in my life at that time? How did it make me feel?* There may be some profound clues as to what you can release based on the answers you receive.

You can also look at parents, aunts, and uncles with the same problem and ask them, *"When did the illness start for you? What was going on in your life at the time (or the year or two before)? How has the illness made you feel?"* Even if you can't or don't want to talk to family members directly, you may be able to put some of the pieces together for yourself. You can also look at broad emotional patterns, common beliefs and behaviors in your extended family.

Remember, as you heal, you may help others in your family to heal, as well. Even if you never say a word, they will experience the new, higher patterns you are creating just from being in your energy. You can use any or all of the exercises in the previous chapters to work with your emotions and beliefs and to access your Inner Healer as you go along. You can also call in your ancestors for support in the following guided meditation.

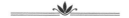

Calling In Your Ancestors

You can work with your ancestors and ask them to help you heal. As you heal, you can help your lineage, in both directions—some people say you can affect seven generations behind you and seven generations beyond you.

1. Close your eyes and watch your breath as it comes in and as it goes out.

2. Allow your mind and heart to become quieter with each breath.

3. When you feel very relaxed, call in all of your ancestors.

4. Very gently bring your awareness to the genetic challenge you are experiencing.

5. Bring in all the family members dealing with this issue. Feel the energy they are carrying. Know that you will still be connected after you resolve this energy into yourself.

6. Release any strong emotion by breathing it in and then breathing out divine love.

7. Ask your ancestors for insights: *Why is your family carrying this challenge? Why are you carrying it? What gifts has it given you? What gifts has it given your other family members?*

8. Ask the ancestors to help you heal yourself and your lineage. Ask them for one practical step you can take.

9. Thank your ancestors and release them.

10. When you are ready, come out of meditation.

11. Follow any guidance you receive.

Do this meditation as often as you like. You may receive different answers and insights each time.

NINE

Medical Mysteries

———— •••————

THINGS LOOK DIFFERENT AS ENERGY

B y the time Sam came to see me, he was feeling desperate. He was a hard-working social worker who was so sick he had had to leave the job where he had been for more than a decade. He had been feeling weak and exhausted for more than two years, and he had lost 12 pounds from his already thin frame. He had first begun feeling sick after a routine colonoscopy, which had shown him to be perfectly healthy. His doctors couldn't find anything wrong. He was dealing with a medical mystery.

Sam is far from alone. Medical mysteries are quite common. Indeed, you might be surprised to know just how many people are dealing with a mystery illness, sometimes going from doctor to doctor, hoping to find help. Yet as mysterious as these illnesses can seem, they can be solved. There is generally an energetic reason for most physical problems. This is good news because when you shift the energy, typically the illness improves or even resolves.

As I did the first healing for Sam, it was clear that he was depleted from having poured tremendous energy into helping the people who came to him for assistance—in particular, children who had been traumatized. I released the energies of exhaustion and his feeling of responsibility. I also ran light for radiant health. Sam returned to his old self after the healing. "What a difference!" he told me, "Thank you so much."

At first, it seemed that one healing had resolved Sam's problem. *That was easy,* I thought to myself, wondering if it would really be that easy, ultimately. In Sam's favor, he had left the job he'd had, so it seemed unlikely that the same problem would reappear. But patterns can be persistent.

Six months later, Sam crashed again. He was exhausted. He had also lost so much weight that when he stepped into my office, he looked unnervingly like a concentration camp prisoner. He was even wearing a grey striped shirt and grey pants that reminded me of a concentration camp uniform.

I don't generally focus on past lives in healing sessions. But the feeling that Sam had perished in a concentration camp in a pervious life became more intense as I laid hands on him and began to run energy. Now I felt I had to mention it even if it wasn't in his belief system.

Fortunately, the concentration camp theme resonated strongly with Sam. While I continued to run energy, he shared that after a spiritual initiation many years earlier, he had had several dreams about being a boy in a concentration camp.

I could see that the little boy Sam had once been died in the camp, feeling that God must not love him if he was being allowed to suffer and die in such a terrible, inhumane way. I shared this impression with Sam and showed the little boy that he was safe, that no harm could come to his soul, and that he had served God deeply by his faith and goodness. I saw that this lifetime had greatly accelerated Sam's spiritual progress; he had remained pure despite the evil around him.

Just a day or two after the healing, Sam went for his appointment with the head of endocrinology at a top teaching hospital. The doctor looked through five years of medical records. "You've had every test," the doctor told Sam. "Nothing shows up. You may just have to accept that this is the way it is for you."

Sam went home feeling utterly dejected. But within the week, as the healing energy began to integrate into his system, Sam began to feel better and better. By the end of the week, he called to tell me he felt completely better. His energy was back, and so were his enthusiasm and joy.

Many aspects of this past incarnation and Sam's current life were integrated in the following weeks through dreams and other guidance. He even came to understand that the colonoscopy, the routine medical examination that had triggered his illness, echoed a less benign "examination" he had endured while in the concentration camp.

Sam's crisis was a mystery medically, but not spiritually. With just two healings, the physical problem resolved. He also developed a much deeper understanding of his life, his past, and his spiritual focus.

MEDICAL MYSTERIES CAN BE SOLVED

More than a few times, someone has come to me with very intense physical problems, and he or she has clearly been suffering, but test after test has been run, scans have been done, and there is no sign of anything wrong. By the time people with such issues find me, they are usually quite distressed.

If you are dealing with your own medical mystery, please don't despair—there is hope for you. Fortunately, a medical diagnosis isn't necessary to heal the problem. You can always work with the underlying energies, whether or not there is a medical explanation for your symptoms.

RECEIVING GUIDANCE

Healings will help a person receive whatever they need, even if what is required is a medical diagnosis. For example,

Celeste was having gastrointestinal issues, but doctors had told her repeatedly that there was nothing wrong with her. But when I tapped into Celeste's energy, I got a very dark, ominous feeling. As I did several healings, I worked to dispel a very dark energy in her field and revitalize her life force, which was very weak. I felt she was facing death.

Finally, I was urgently guided to ask: *Do you have life insurance?* That was the question I heard as *Spirit* whispered in my ear. I ignored it. I heard it again, more insistently. Again I ignored the spirit voice, though it was now even more emphatic.

Finally, after *Spirit* prodded me again, I conveyed the question to Celeste. "What kind of question is that?" she replied, furious. However, the question galvanized Celeste to insist on further testing from her doctors. Finally, they found her cancer. Celeste had stage IIIC cancer of the fallopian tubes. That question about life insurance probably saved her life.

Celeste received healings, chemotherapy, and homeopathy. Her tumors shrank. She then had surgery. Because her tumors had shrunk so significantly by then, her surgeon was able to spare her rectum and colon, making her surgery far less devastating and life altering than originally expected.

Based on her surgeon's tempered comments right after surgery, I don't think Celeste's doctors believed she would survive long term. But I am happy to report that Celeste has now been cancer-free for close to a decade.

TERRIBLE SYMPTOMS, BUT NO PHYSICAL CAUSE

Occasionally someone will come to me for healing who is suffering from terrible physical symptoms, having had every test in the book, and there will truly be nothing "physically" wrong. I consider these people lucky, although they are often desperate for a "real" diagnosis. They are lucky because the energetic problem has not manifested in a physical ailment—or at least, not yet.

Helen, for example, had severe gastrointestinal pain. She was desperate and wished madly for a diagnosis, but she never got one. From my perspective, the issue was an energy imbalance. She was just so tense and such a perfectionist that her system was in a constant state of distress. As we did healings, she had more and more days when she felt better, but she stopped having healings before her symptoms completely resolved. It was too painful for her to let go of her vision of the world, of her need to keep things picture-perfect, even though it was making her sick.

IDIOPATHIC ILLNESS

Another type of medical mystery encompasses the many disorders deemed "idiopathic" by doctors. They appear mysteriously, and they may have names, like "macular degeneration," but there is no medical explanation for why they occur—they just do. Many autoimmune diseases fall into this category. The energy of these illnesses and disorders can be worked with and healed.

As you can see, there are as many different answers to medical mysteries as there are mysteries: Each case is unique. But healing will almost always shed light and bring relief.

You can work with the energy of these issues. Try the exercises in the previous chapters to see what your Inner Healer will tell you and help you to release. You can also try the guided meditation on the following page, "Working with Your Mystery Illness."

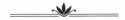

Working With Your Mystery Illness

You can unravel the mysteries of your illness.

1. Close your eyes and watch your breath as it comes in and as it goes out.

2. Allow your mind and heart to become quieter with each breath.

3. When you feel very relaxed, call in the light and divine love. If you wish, you can also call in your Inner Healer or a spiritual master or archangel.

4. Very gently bring your awareness to your mystery illness.

5. Identify one "theme" your illness expresses. For instance, an autoimmune disease might be about the body attacking itself. Macular degeneration might be about being afraid to see something in your life.

6. Ask your Inner Healer to show you how that theme may be expressing itself in other areas of your life. For instance, if you are suffering from an autoimmune disease, do you attack yourself, or does someone in your life attack you? If you have something like macular degeneration, is there something you have been afraid to look at?

7. Set your intention to clear this theme in your day-to-day life. Ask your Inner Healer for one action you can take right now.

8. When you are ready, thank the light and your Inner Healer or any master or archangel you called in. Gently come out of meditation.

9. Follow the guidance you have received as you go about your life.

10. Notice what unfolds.

Do this meditation as often as you like.

TEN

Accidents and Injuries

———— • • ————

WORKING WITH THE MATRIX

Rebecca had been in a serious car accident. Both knees were broken. On her right leg, the femur and the tibia, the bones that connect to the knee plate, were also broken, and her right ankle had been badly dislocated.

Her son called me to ask for help the day after the accident. I started the healing immediately. The sooner you can begin adding healing light to a traumatic injury, the faster the healing process will be and the more likely it is that everything will heal perfectly, without lingering problems or pain.

Energy, at the most basic level, is life force. We can use our energy to help jump-start someone else. In principle, it's similar to jump-starting a dying battery in a car, but a healer draws on the universal energy field so she doesn't completely drain her own "battery." When you add extra energy to someone, his or her body will use it to speed up the healing process. You can also repair any energy channels that have been disrupted

I could tell immediately that Rebecca's right leg needed my focus the most. Through a deep resonance, I could feel the searing pain in her knee as if it was in my own body, even though I was working long distance. I knew the healing light might make the difference as to whether Rebecca's leg healed completely or not. I was worried that without healing light, that leg might not be normal again.

That first week I did several healings. Then Rebecca and I worked together regularly for several more weeks. Each time, her body insisted that I focus mostly on her right leg. I also gave light to all of her broken bones, including her sternum and collarbone, and worked on releasing the fear and emotional trauma caused by the impact.

I also worked on releasing some negative energies that I saw had contributed to the accident. At the time of the accident, Rebecca was involved in a business litigation with a very difficult person who had a strong ill intent aimed at her. Rebecca hadn't caused the accident in any way. A car going in the opposite direction had come into Rebecca's lane. But I felt that her legal adversary's bad intentions had affected the universal field around her.

Rebecca healed quickly. Amazingly, when the doctors took her casts off, it was the right leg, which had been so badly damaged, that she was allowed to stand on and bend first.

When she had regained her strength and the use of her legs, she moved quickly to settle the legal case. It meant accepting a smaller settlement than she might have won in court. But she decided to enjoy her precious life instead of engaging with this dark force any further.

THE LIVING MATRIX

Our bodies are amazing, mysterious, and mystical; it's better than sci-fi. Take the living matrix upon which everything grows, even your cells. You have a matrix—or web—of energy interpenetrating your body. (Think of the Spiderman character.) This matrix feeds energy to each and every cell. When there's a trauma to the body, that living matrix is disrupted.

We can easily repair that matrix so as to heal more quickly and completely. When the energy lines are repaired so that they are complete and radiant, the body can heal properly, following the underlying energy pattern. That is one of the things I did to help Rebecca. The sooner you can start adding light, the better the result will be. In fact, minor injuries can sometimes disappear if healing energy is applied immediately, before the body has had time to fully register the injury or allow it to settle in. Major injuries can be significantly ameliorated.

I learned this while I was still a journalist investigating healing. One of the healers I was interviewing, Dani, told me that she had had a bad knock to her head that left her with a gash, as well. A friend, also a healer, ran energy through the matrix right after the accident. The gash disappeared in just hours—along with all the discomfort in Dani's head. When she arrived the next day at the hospital to get a scan of her head just to be safe, they looked at her as if she were crazy; there was no sign of any injury at all.

A FINGER CAUGHT IN A CAR DOOR

I soon got a chance to try this out myself. I was visiting with friends when a car-pooling mom was dropping off my friend's child. The automatic door of the van closed on another boy's finger. The boy was howling in pain when he was brought into the house.

While the other adults debated in a panic about whether to rush the boy to the emergency room or call his parents first, I sat down next to the boy and began running energy into his injured finger, which was already swelling badly.

In ten minutes, the boy had calmed down. Everyone in the room got very quiet because they could feel the energy. After twenty minutes, the boy's finger looked normal once again. He announced that he wanted to go out and play. He was healed.

A BAD CUT

A few years later, it was my turn: I cut my finger in the kitchen of my meditation center. It was a deep cut, and there was a great deal of blood. A doctor who happened to be there insisted that I go to the emergency room immediately. As I waited to be seen, I worked on healing the lines of energy, the matrix on which the cells grow. When the triage nurse unwrapped my bandages, she gave me an odd look.

"Is it very bad?" I asked.

"No," she replied. "It's already closed up."

I took a look at my finger. Indeed, the skin had knitted itself back together. Ever since, I've wished that there was a healer in every ambulance and emergency room. Maybe someday.

REPAIRING BONES

Andy

Bones are very responsive to healing light. Patty, one of my advanced students, demonstrated this recently. She had been transmitting radiant light to a teenager named Andy for about a year, ever since Andy had broken his spinal column in a diving accident and become a quadriplegic. Nevertheless, he had continued to hang out with his friends, who were very committed to him.

Around the time Patty was working on Andy, he went to an amusement park with his friends. His legs swelled up on the way home, so they took him to a doctor who diagnosed broken knees. (Andy hadn't had his legs strapped in during the rides.) Patty began working on Andy's knees that day.

When Andy was reexamined three weeks after breaking his knees, the doctor found they were almost completely healed. The doctor concluded that Andy must have broken his knees weeks or months earlier than everyone had believed—broken knees don't heal that rapidly, he told them.

I encouraged Patty to keep working on Andy's spine. Nerve damage is much more difficult to heal than bones, and nerves are also much slower to regenerate, but some healing could still occur. Also, whatever happened with Andy's spine, the healings were clearly helping him to navigate socially and emotionally despite the immobilizing injury.

Peggy

Bones are surprisingly easy to work with, considering how solid they seem. When Peggy came to me for help, her arm was in a cast, broken from a recent fall, and she was quite worried. Her doctors wanted to operate and set a pin in her bone to make sure it healed properly. Peggy didn't want the operation. I ran a lot of energy into Peggy's arm, knowing that if she needed the operation as well as the healing, she would be guided by the energy.

Over the course of the session, Peggy's pain level ratcheted up, but as I explained to her, it wasn't that the healing was causing pain. The energy I was transmitting was simply bringing awareness to what was there. The energy would also help the bone heal rapidly and ideally. Peggy was in pain for most of a week, but her bone healed perfectly.

HOLDING THE LIGHT FOR YOURSELF AND OTHERS

You can work on healing the energy matrix whenever there's been a physical injury and it will support the healing process. You can try the guided meditation, "Healing The Matrix," on the next page to help yourself or someone you love.

We can also always hold light for others. Another way to do that is to work with the meditation, "Healing Physical Trauma," at the end of this chapter.

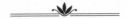

Healing the Matrix

We can help our bodies heal from trauma by adding light and repairing the living matrix.

1. Close your eyes and watch your breath as it comes in and as it goes out.

2. With each breath, let yourself go deeper.

3. When you feel very relaxed, call in the light and divine love. Also call in your Inner Healer, the part of you that knows exactly what you need to heal.

4. Bring into your awareness the part of your body you want to heal.

5. Visualize radiant light in this area.

6. Imagine that there is an energy grid throughout this area.

7. You may think of a tic-tac-toe board with white lines and then make it three-dimensional. It's okay if you think you are imagining it.

8. See where the lines could be finer or brighter and add more light.

9. There may be places where the lines are broken or missing, or places where they are tangled. With your intention, imagine that these lines are all repaired. The gridwork is now perfect. You can do this purely in your mind or right above the physical body where the trauma is, using a finger to trace the energy lines.

10. When you feel the grid is now perfect, thank this part of your body. Thank your Inner Healer and any guides or masters you have called in.

Do this healing meditation regularly to help you heal from a physical trauma.

TRAUMATIC HEAD INJURY

One of the most dramatic recoveries from traumatic injury in which I've participated involved 8-year-old Neil, who was playing hide-and-seek on the roof of his building when he tripped and fell three stories. When the paramedics reached him, blood was leaking out of one of his ears, and they didn't think he was going to make it. By the time family friends called me a day later, Neil was lying in a coma in a hospital, barely hanging on. He was so fragile that his doctors weren't allowing anyone except his parents to see him. Fortunately, healing energy is not bound by time and space, doors and walls, or hospital routines.

I went into a deep state and connected with Neil soul to soul. When I reached him, his energy field was frozen in panic and shock. I held him ever so gently in the highest, most soothing light. It took about two hours before he began to relax, but eventually Neil let his heart come to rest in my heart. When his energy finally began to flow, I felt confident that he would live.

Once Neil had calmed down, I gently turned my awareness to his brain. There was so much pain in his head that the gentlest touch of energy—even at a distance—caused him to panic all over again. I had to work very gently and slowly to calm him down and add healing light to his head. Then I restructured the energy grid on which his brain cells grew.

Very slowly, the enormous pressure and pain in his head began to subside—and with it his panic. During the next week, Neil was indeed extremely agitated. This was because the panic I had unraveled from his energy field was now releasing from his system. As he began to emerge from his coma, his doctors put him into an induced coma to keep him as still as possible.

After two weeks, Neil emerged from the medically induced coma and was soon talking, laughing, and smiling. Within a matter of weeks the hospital released him, and although he was still fragile, he went home. His doctors considered his recovery a miracle.

A COLICKY BABY

Healings can often be effective even months or years after a trauma, when pain or discomfort persist.

Samantha called me because her 4-month-old baby girl, Callie, had been colicky since birth. In addition, Callie had chronic intestinal problems and couldn't drink her mother's milk, which was upsetting both mother and baby.

Samantha told me that her pregnancy had been normal. When I questioned her more thoroughly, she mentioned that a few weeks before giving birth, she had been in a car accident. She and the baby had been fine according to the doctors. However, the close call had shaken Samantha terribly.

When I did the healing, I saw that the baby was still in a state of shock. I released her fear and transmitted healing light to her intestines to soothe them. I also strengthened the bond between baby and mother. A week later, Samantha told me that Callie was like a different child: "She's not perfect, but the difference is like night and day," she said. Callie was even able to nurse at her breast.

ACCIDENTS AREN'T ALWAYS "ACCIDENTAL"

There is often a deep symbology behind an accident. Or, to put it another way, injuries often express energies that were present at the time of the accident. When you clear that energy, the body can heal more completely and a person's life can shift for the better.

It never ceases to amaze me how deeply our souls talk to us through our bodies, even when the injury is from an accident. Once I was in a social setting with a man named Steven, who had a broken wrist. I offered to run a little energy so his bone would knit together faster.

I was thinking that a little healing light would simply accelerate the physical repair. But suddenly, as the energy began to run, I was in touch with the emotional pain that made this man want to dominate others. I could tell Steven was conscious of it, too. He began to cry as he shared with me how he had tried to force his horse's will. In protest, the horse had thrown him. A few months earlier, he added, the horse had thrown him for the same reason, that time dislocating his shoulder.

His epiphany was so powerful that I sensed it could potentially change the way he treated others in the future. That alone would change his life.

CERVICAL DISC REPAIR

Gina, a nurse, had slipped and fallen in the hospital where she worked. In our first session, I could see this had not really been an accident. She had not been happy in her job for a long time. The "accident" was her soul's way of getting her out of the job.

The specific nature of the injury was also informative. Gina had damaged the disc in her spine between the C4 and C5 vertebrae. This told me that she was having issues between her heart (fourth chakra) and her speech (fifth chakra). As I continued to run energy, her body showed me that she was expressing pain in her heart with sharp words.

As we worked together over several months, healing saints began visiting Gina in dreams and waking visions. She began studying guided imagery and awakened her light body. A year into her healing journey, Gina's MRI pictures showed a physical improvement in her spinal column at the location of the injured disc, and yet the disc itself had not gotten better. Gina decided to have surgery to replace her damaged disc with an artificial one. In a guided-imagery session, she saw that the surgeon she had chosen was part of her healing path, and this gave her the confidence to go ahead.

In a long-distance session, I transmitted light to Gina during her surgery. I saw that the new artificial disc would cushion her words as she began to speak her truth.

Soon after her surgery, Gina's husband fell ill. She met the challenge valiantly. Serving as a healer and caretaker, she turned into a saint before my eyes with her kindness, compassion and selfless devotion.

A TWISTED ANKLE

Even something as simple as a twisted ankle can have deep meaning. Stephanie called me from the emergency room hours after she had tripped over her dog, tearing ligaments in her right ankle and breaking her left knee. She also mentioned in almost the same breath that she had run into her former beau at a party the night before. It was clear to her that he still loved her and she was upset that he was with another woman. I told Stephanie that I would work on everything, as the physical and emotional issues were very likely related.

Although the knee sounded like the more challenging problem, as I tuned in and transmitted healing energy, it was her ankle that was throbbing terribly. I ran many high frequencies to help her ankle. Then I worked on her knee to help the bone fracture heal. I saw that Stephanie had lost her emotional balance after seeing her ex, and this had led her to lose her physical balance. I held light for her heartache to heal. We did a second healing a few days later and then another session a week or so after that. By then, the pain in Stephanie's ankle had subsided quite a bit.

The doctor had told Stephanie that the ankle sprain was so bad it would take more than two months to heal, but she was out of a brace in two weeks. The doctor had expected her knee to take six months to heal, but after a month he declared that it was healing wonderfully. She was out of the full brace within six weeks.

Stephanie was grateful to be back on her feet so quickly. She made her peace with her breakup and went on to have a very productive time in her life and work.

ACCIDENTS CAN GUIDE US

Accidents happen when you least expect them. Maybe you're tired or not paying attention, or perhaps you have other things on your mind. An accident gets your attention. It requires your focus.

Even a simple injury can be a message from your soul. When you have an injury, it's important to ask yourself: *What is the symbology? What is my soul trying to tell me?* When we learn what our souls want for us, we know the right path forward. There is nothing more fulfilling, comforting and empowering than being in alignment with your soul.

A CRACKED ELBOW

Friends of mine were visiting me in Los Angeles when Susie, the wife, leaned backward as she got out of my car. I heard a huge cracking sound as her husband slammed the rear door shut—somehow, Susie's elbow had gotten caught in the door. She was reeling from the pain and looked nauseated. I took her into the house and immediately began running energy, though I hadn't even eaten breakfast yet.

As I did the healing, the first thing I saw was that Susie was weary to the bone; she was working too hard at something she no longer loved. I heard that if she did not make a change, she could get very sick. Second, I saw that my own impatience had contributed to the accident. I had been too wound up about getting everything done and taking care of my guests to be as gracious and present as I would have liked to be. I apologized for this as I ran the energy. Within half an hour, all of the pain and swelling was gone. By the end of the day, it was as if the accident had never happened.

As the weeks unfolded, Susie found new ways to open to her artistic and spiritual gifts so that she would be replenished. I can't say that it was all because of the healing, but I believe the energy made the shift a little easier.

IT'S NEVER TOO LATE FOR HEALING

I've cleared pain from injuries that happened years, even decades, earlier. Although the pain may seem entirely physical, it has been my experience that when the soul issues are addressed, even after many years, the pain will diminish or even completely disappear. The pain is a marker for a soul issue that is crying out to be resolved.

Take the case of Sally, who had shattered her leg and arm in a motorcycle accident a dozen years earlier. The arm had healed, but she still had terrible, disabling pain in her leg. I had no idea what her body would tell me or even whether it would have anything to say. As soon as I began running energy, however, her leg began to talk to me. It revealed to me that Sally had a fear of moving forward in life. *Ah,* I thought to myself. *Yes, that's exactly what happened.* Her motorcycle's brakes had locked, preventing her from moving forward, and as a result she had flown over the handlebars.

The accident had happened on the night that Sally was writing her medical school applications. Because of the ongoing pain from her injured leg as the result of the accident, she ultimately decided to get a nursing degree instead of pursuing her dream. As I worked, I could feel her wistfulness. "You know, maybe you still want to go to medical school," I said.

"I'm 40. But I still think about it," she told me.

"Well, the time will pass anyway," I said.

We talked about the ways she could make her dream happen. "Maybe this isn't a detour," I continued, still reading the energy. "Sometimes people are slow-cooked," I said. "You know how things can take on a richness that way?" She lit up. She had never looked at her situation this way.

Her leg had one other message. It didn't like the rod holding the bones in place. "It helped in the initial healing because the bones were in so many pieces," she told me. "But maybe because my leg bones never had to bear all of their own weight, they didn't heal completely. I will have to contemplate this."

I felt we had made some progress during the session. Only time will tell what Sally will end up doing, but understanding the body symbology can open the door to immense healing.

PERSISTENT PAIN

Henry's problem started in college, when he suffered a fairly minor knee injury playing soccer. Surgery was suggested to fix the injury. When that surgery didn't work, he went for another surgery. He eventually underwent a series of surgeries but his leg bothered him more with each surgery and became non functional.

I only wish Henry could have found a healer back when he was still in school. If he had, I believe his life could have taken a different path. Even now, he could still have healed many issues related to the leg and greatly improved the quality of his life along with his emotional state. He tried one healing, but he didn't feel that this was his path.

My suggestion is that if you have a persistent problem, you should get to the root cause so you can truly heal. Your whole life will be better.

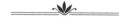

Healing Physical Trauma

Here's a simple, effective method for holding light for others to alleviate injuries and trauma. You do not have to be in the same room as the person for whom you are holding light.

1. Close your eyes and watch your breath as it comes in and as it goes out.

2. With each breath, drop more deeply into your inner self, letting go of any thoughts, and allowing the breath to slow and expand.

3. When you feel very relaxed, call in the light and divine love and your Inner Healer. If you wish, you can also call in a spiritual master or archangel.

4. If it is medically safe, very gently place your hands on the injury. Otherwise, you can place your hands above the injury. You can also simply stand nearby and hold an intention to transmit light. If you are in a separate location, imagine you are holding your hands on the injury.

5. Set an intention for peace and radiant health. Imagine that the light in your heart is traveling down your hands and into the injured area. You may also silently repeat the Lord's Prayer or your own personal favorite prayer.

6. Hold this beautiful energy transmission for at least 10 minutes or for as long as you feel comfortable.

7. Silently thank the light, the person you have been healing, your Inner Healer and any master or archangel you called in. You can now release your hands.

You can do this healing meditation regularly until the injury is resolved.

ELEVEN

Surgery

———— •••• ————

PREPARING AND HEALING

I wish everyone here could receive an energy treatment," said the nurse in charge of the recovery room at New York City's Memorial Sloan Kettering Cancer Center, one of the top cancer hospitals in the country. She gestured around the grim room where people lay absorbed in a mixture of pain and mind-numbing drugs amid the blips and humming of monitors.

"It would cut down on the suffering and the amount of meds we have to use," she continued, drawing a curtain around the bed where I sat with Celeste, who had just had major surgery to remove cancer of the fallopian tubes that had spread to several other organs and areas.

Celeste was pale and lifeless, but keenly aware of intense pain. I couldn't wait to begin running energy for her. I knew that it would help her feel better. By the time Celeste's fallopian tube cancer had been discovered it was classified as stage IIIC. Who knows if it even would have been found in time to save Celeste without the healings we did. (See Chapter 9: "Medical Mysteries" for more details.)

IN THE RECOVERY ROOM

Now all of that medical treatment was behind her. Directly after her surgery I ran energy for Celeste for more than an hour. As I worked, I ran very high frequencies of energy to lift the trauma, pain, and anesthesia and replace it all with radiant light. At first, I could feel all of the toxins and trauma, almost as if they were in my body. I knew we were making progress as her nausea and distress began to subside. It was a relief for both of us.

I then reconnected all of the lines of energy on which the cells and organs grow. That way everything could heal properly. Finally, I turned my energy to comforting her at a soul level so that she would know, physically and spiritually, that she was safe. Once her system was soothed and her energy developed a good flow, she could begin to heal.

Celeste was practically a different person when I said good-bye for the night. Overall, she made a great recovery. Blood tests showed that her cancer markers had returned to normal immediately after surgery. Her oncologist told her not to get her hopes up, but she has been completely cancer-free for nearly a decade now.

ADD LIGHT BEFORE AND AFTER SURGERY

If you are facing surgery, it is good to add healing light both before and after your operation. Before the surgery, it will help things go as smoothly and successfully as possible. Afterward, you can greatly accelerate the healing process by repairing the energy matrix and generally restoring your health and vitality.

When I work with someone who is facing surgery, I am always looking to create the highest possible flow and add the most possible light to his or her energy. You can do this, too, when preparing yourself or a loved one for surgery. With the transmission of healing light before and after surgery, I've seen women wake from mastectomies without pain, and surgeons comment on how little blood loss there was during complex, life-threatening operations.

A WHIPPLE PROCEDURE

Henrietta had pancreatic cancer and was facing extensive abdominal surgery, known as a Whipple Procedure, which would take out part of her digestive system. When we started working together, Henrietta, in her 70s was quite discouraged about her health. Her energy was gray and stagnant. It did not move that much in the first healing. The heavy effects of the illness and her fear around the surgery had taken their toll on her energy.

Fortunately, Henrietta asked for more healings. We did four or five more sessions leading up to her surgery. The energy kept building until, a few days before her surgery, it had become ecstatic and extraordinarily dynamic. There was simply an exciting flow to the energy that was enjoyable for me to experience. Her energy could dance with my energy, and I knew as a result the surgery would have the best of all possible outcomes.

Indeed, the surgery went remarkably well. The surgeon had to do less cutting than expected, and there was almost no bleeding—a remarkable fact, as the surgeon noted to Henrietta and her family. When the pathology report came back, it turned out that Henrietta's cancer was less aggressive than the doctors had originally thought and her prognosis was much better than they had believed it would be.

In the days after her surgery I continued to do healings for Henrietta to help repair her energy matrix and restore her vitality. She was off painkillers in almost no time. Ten days after her operation, her surgeons said that she was a month ahead of schedule in her recovery.

Henrietta had experienced the miracle of great energy flow. In her doctors' view, she made a remarkable recovery from her surgery. She was able to eat a relatively normal diet. Pleased with her progress, she soon stopped having healings. She was cancer-free for more than a year. When her vitality began to ebb again, her doctors diagnosed her with a recurrence of a lymphoma that she had successfully battled decades earlier. This time she did not seek medical treatment or healings and she passed peacefully.

CREATING EASE AND GRACE

You don't have to be an expert at transmitting energy to add light to your own surgery. Adding light is always beneficial. It brings things to a higher order. You can use the guided meditations, "Adding Light Before Surgery" and "Recovering From Surgery," towards the end of this chapter.

A HIP REPLACEMENT

Lynn, a nurse who was studying energy medicine with me, needed a hip replacement. She was anxious about the surgery, having had several previous surgeries that had not gone well. With my encouragement, she prepared herself by transmitting light to her hip, to the operating room, and to her surgeon in advance.

While I am confident that adding light brings everything to the highest place, I never know in advance exactly how that will look. In Lynn's case, I had a front-row seat when I visited her in the hospital the day after her surgery. "I have less pain now than before the surgery," she marveled as she got out of her hospital bed and walked to the bathroom by herself.

A few minutes later, Lynn's surgeon came into the room to check on her, and he was delighted—and surprised—that Lynn was walking around. He shared a bit about the surgery itself because it had been so special, even for him.

"Usually you have one or two doctors doing this kind of surgery," he told Lynn proudly, "but one of the other surgeons was going to play golf with us in the afternoon, so he joined us in the operating room. You had three top orthopedic surgeons working on you. Each one of us personally checked the alignment of your hip. One of those surgeons was even working for free. You know, that never happens." Lynn and I exchanged glances. Pleased with how everything had turned out, her doctor sauntered happily out of the room.

A PANCREATIC CYST

Andrea's operation also went more smoothly than expected, with a terrific outcome. Her doctors had discovered a cyst on her pancreas. "It's probably benign," she told me as she sat across from me in my office, "but they have to make sure, so I have to have an operation."

I wasn't surprised that if Andrea had a medical problem, it was showing up in her abdominal area. Whenever I did a healing with Andrea, that area lit up as her "hot spot." She had an energetic knot there; it's where she stored her stress. Regularly scheduled healings might have dissolved it, but she could barely make time for a healing even every other month. Andrea was one of the busiest people I knew, juggling her high-powered career; marriage to a wonderful, successful man; and being a devoted mom to three sweet kids.

The cyst was small, but in order to remove it, Andrea's surgeon said he would probably also have to remove her spleen and part of her pancreas. "The worst of it is, I'll probably have a big vertical scar up and down my abdomen," Andrea said. "So long as I'm healthy, that's OK, I guess." She paused. "What can you do to help?"

I did a healing for Andrea a week before the surgery and a second healing the night before the operation. I held light for the highest outcome and added light to the surgeon, his hands, and the operating room. I also transmitted healing light to Andrea's abdomen so that the surgery would be as simple and noninvasive as possible and she would recover quickly. By the time I closed the second session, I had a very good feeling. The next morning, I dedicated my morning prayers to Andrea.

Andrea's operation took longer than expected, but the surgeon was able to do the procedure with a laparoscope, something he hadn't expected to be possible. He made just the tiniest incision and relied on a video probe to guide the tools while they were inside her abdomen, leaving her spleen and pancreas intact.

"He seemed so proud, like he had really done a terrific job," Andrea told me when we talked the next day. Best of all, Andrea's cyst turned out to be benign.

AFTER SURGERY

The first time I did a healing for someone directly after surgery, I didn't know what to expect. Doctors had put a pin in Margaret's thighbone, which was weakened from cancer. When I sat with her in the recovery room, I ran light into the area of the operation and restructured the matrix, but I also sensed a deep loneliness, and I released it.

"I don't know what you did," she told me afterward, "but I didn't have any pain."

I thought it was a quirk that Margaret reported a total lack of pain, but I have since found that this can be one effect of healing light after surgery.

A DOUBLE MASTECTOMY

Lydia came to see me after she was diagnosed with a tiny ductal carcinoma in situ in her breast. Under normal circumstances, she would have had a lumpectomy. However, she had a family history of breast cancer. As unusual as it sounds, her father had died of breast cancer. Therefore, her doctors recommended a double mastectomy.

I worked with Lydia before the surgery to prepare her. Both she and her health care practitioners were surprised at how little pain she had after her surgery.

I continued to do healings after the surgery to provide ongoing support. While Lydia was having her chest wall expanded to accommodate her new implants, she told me, "They asked me if I was having any pain. They seemed surprised that I was doing so well."

Lydia noticed an unexpected side effect of the healings as well: "The back pain I've had for years is also so much better than it has ever been. I have less pain now than when I was taking painkillers to control the pain."

Lydia's experience isn't all that unusual. Again and again, I've seen that healing light can reduce and sometimes even eliminate postsurgical pain. Nevertheless, I was still surprised when Lee Anne, in her late 70s, reported a lack of pain after a mastectomy. Again, I did healings before and after her surgery, and she was thrilled to sail through it.

CRISIS IN THE OPERATING ROOM

Selena, who studied energy healing with me, scheduled a surgery to realign her jaw, which she thought would help the flow of energy into her head and alleviate her constant headaches. She had to have her jaw broken in four different places and reset, six hours of major surgery. We worked as a team on her surgery and recovery. Instead of having a healing before her surgery, Selena wanted me to start the healing process as soon as she got into the recovery room. It was as if some part of her knew in advance that she would be in critical need of help.

I sat in the waiting room for quite a long time. Finally, when I inquired after her, the attendant told me that Selena was too unstable for visitors. I knew then that something was terribly wrong, and I began a long-distance healing immediately, while still sitting in the waiting room. As soon as I touched in, I saw that Selena's heart was agitated and that she was in a critical state, on the verge of death.

I ran energy into her heart to stabilize her. (Much later, her doctors told me that Selena had stopped breathing after the surgery and they had had trouble stabilizing her.) I also brought in the souls of her four children and showed Selena how important it was for her to continue to serve as their mother. After close to an hour, Selena finally relaxed, and her heart stabilized. I was not at all surprised when, minutes later, her doctors paged me and said I could go and see her.

In the recovery room, I did several hours of energy work with Selena to calm her traumatized body and accelerate her healing process. I came back the next morning and worked with her again. I encouraged Selena to continue running energy into her own jaw on a daily, even hourly, basis.

Selena healed easily. She had a brief surgical infection, but much to her doctor's amazement, she was able to knock it out. After one follow-up exam, she reported, "There was absolutely no sign that there was ever an infection. No drainage area, no puffiness, no discoloration, no tenderness—and the doctor was really pushing all around. He said it just doesn't happen like this, completely new and fresh with no sign of anything whatsoever. He said he's a believer now [in the healing energy] and to keep it up. He kept talking about it. He was amazed."

Selena was completely healed in a few months, and with her jaw straightened out, she looked great and felt much better.

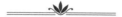

Adding Light Before Surgery

It's always a good idea to add light before going in for any surgery. I have seen many surgeries go better than expected when light is added. To help someone facing surgery:

1. Close your eyes and focus on your breath as it comes in and as it goes out.

2. Allow yourself to go deeper with each breath.

3. When you feel very relaxed, call in the light and your Inner Healer and if you wish, a healing master or archangel.

4. Imagine the operating room and the surgeon bathed in radiant light.

5. See the person who is going to have the surgery, whether it is you or a loved one, bathed in light.

6. Add light to the area of the body where the surgery will be. In your mind's eye, see the energy matrix that underlies the body and make it a perfect 3D grid.

7. Silently thank the light and your Inner Healer along with the surgeons and nurses, and any masters or archangels you called in. Gently come out of meditation.

A PRECANCEROUS CERVIX

Surgery works on physical problems, and often it's essential. But if the underlying root causes of the problem are not addressed, surgery may not totally repair the problem, or an operation may be more arduous than it would be normally. When we clear and harmonize the underlying energy, the surgery can have the highest flow and best outcome possible.

Christine, a very attractive, bubbly career woman, came to me for a session just before she was to have surgery on her cervix, where her doctor had found a collection of precancerous cells. He warned her that the surgery would be hard on her cervix and that she would require a long healing period.

When I laid hands on Christine, I saw that the irregular cells growing in her cervix were connected to her sexual involvement with men who were not truly loving or committed. As I ran energy, I saw that she had never had a happy ending to any of her romantic relationships, and the pain her soul had endured had been deep. I helped release this dark, toxic energy from her body, and it seemed to dissipate in waves. "My God, I can feel the energy vibrating inside of me," she exclaimed at one point.

Her surgery turned out to be far less invasive than her doctor had predicted. In my view, this was because the healing had dissipated the worst of the dark energy and already shifted the matrix for her cervix's physical health. Christine made a rapid recovery.

MULTIPLE SURGERIES, LINGERING PAIN

Sometimes surgery leads to more surgeries in the same area, which could be because of ongoing pain that theoretically should have been resolved. In other cases, a person gets one new crisis after another in the same area of the body, requiring repeated surgeries. Usually this type of ongoing trauma indicates that the underlying energetic issues have not been adequately addressed.

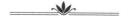

Recovering From Surgery

We can help our bodies heal after surgery by adding light and repairing the living matrix. You can also combine this meditation with the "Listening to Your Body" meditation.

1. Close your eyes and watch your breath as it comes in and as it goes out.

2. With each breath, let go of any thoughts and let yourself go deeper. Feel your breath naturally slow and expand.

3. When you feel very relaxed, call in the light and your Inner Healer.

4. Call up in your mind's eye the area of your body where you had surgery. Imagine or visualize radiant light in this area.

6. See (or imagine) the energy grid for this area. See where the lines could be finer or brighter. Add light. With your intention, imagine that these lines are all repaired. The grid work is now perfect.

7 . Silently thank the light and your Inner Healer. Gently come out of meditation..

Do this healing meditation regularly to heal from surgery.

Lauren, a petite, neat, well-dressed mother of four grown children, was a textbook example of ongoing postsurgical trouble. I met her when she came to a talk I gave in a small town outside of New York City shortly after my first book was published. When I asked for a volunteer for a healing demonstration, she raised her hand before anyone else.

Lauren looked great, but her appearance belied the reality. Her problem had begun decades earlier with an obstruction in her bowel, which doctors had tried to alleviate through surgery. She had developed adhesions after the surgery and was in constant pain. She had tried everything, but nothing seemed to help.

As Lauren lay down on the healing table, I slowly moved my hands along key energy points on her body. Soon our hearts began to beat in rhythm with each other. Her breathing became very slow and regular, as if she were asleep. We had come into resonance.

As I held my hands on Lauren's pelvis, her body began to show me the true cause of her pain. I saw how early religious teachings had caused her to suppress her sexuality even as a little girl. Eventually she had constricted all of the energy in her pelvic area. I began to release the contraction and showed Lauren that her energy was divine.

Lauren woke feeling deliciously calm. A few weeks later, she called to tell me how, after our session, she had decided it was time to release the guilt she still felt about a relationship from 30 years earlier that had ended with an abortion. A few days after the healing, she sought the counsel of a priest. The guilt, loss, and sadness finally lifted, and she was more comfortable physically.

TWELVE

Seven Essentials for Healing

———— • • • ————

BE STILL, AND KNOW THAT I AM GOD

—PSALM 46:10, THE BIBLE

Inside each of us is a divine light. It is the source of infinite love and wisdom. When we connect to our innermost Self, we receive support and guidance, ease and grace. Indeed, one of the most wonderful healing tools we have at our disposal involves going within. As Jesus, one of the great spiritual teachers in history, taught, "The Kingdom of God is within you."

If you find it hard to go inward, don't give up. You can do it, and it will be worth the effort and focus many times over. It truly helps if you can accept whatever pain you are experiencing, instead of fighting it. Simply connect to the pain by going within, and be present with it. You may see it soften, or even dissolve. Or you will be guided on your next steps.

The following are a few tools to help you connect to the deepest, wisest part of your being and support you on your healing journey. These practices can be used again and again for almost anything you want to heal. I offer them to people who come to me for healing support, and I also use them for myself. They are easy, but powerful and transformative. It is good to review and work with them as often as you are drawn to do so. I highly recommend that you work with these practices while doing the guided meditations in this book.

HAVE A CLEAR INTENTION

Whatever you want to accomplish, it's always a good idea to set a clear intention. *What do you want to heal? What are you trying to create in your life?* A healing journey is like any other journey. It's important to have a goal, to know where you want to go. Then set that goal as your intention.

Intention is a powerful force. It exists and operates at the causal level of your being, a deeper level than your thoughts and feelings. Your intentions (and your desires) direct your energy and the energy of the universal field. Everything you do starts with an intention or desire, whether you are conscious of the intent or desire, or not.

When you harness the power of intention in a conscious way, your life enters a different domain. After all, you are harnessing the energies of the universe to work with you in a focused and coherent way. You will see results.

Intention isn't a demanding, willful energy. Rather, it is a quiet force, like the rudder on a boat. You set your intention, and then you let things happen. You take the actions that you need to take. But you allow things to unfold. You can work hard. But you don't have to struggle or push. When things don't go your way, you trust that there is a higher reason. There is some other way that will be better and easier to get you to your goal.

Sometimes as we go along our path, guided by a clear intention, we will come across obstacles. This is often because we haven't cleared some belief or thought. The challenge gives us the opportunity to clear our unconscious so we can actually reach our goal in the highest way.

Intention is a beautiful force to harness with everything you do. On the following pages I offer some tips for working with intention and a guided meditation.

Tips for Working with Intention

* **Always frame your intention in a positive way.** For example, hold an intention for radiant health rather than not to be sick. You can also hold an intention for radiant health and to heal any illness and all the underlying issues. Radiant health, inner peace, and clarity are very high intentions. They are simple and can take you a very long way. I use them for myself, too.

* **Refine your intentions as you go.** You may find that the overall goal of radiant health is a good one for you. But in the short term you may have more specific intentions that are a subset of your global intention, such as to be able to sleep at night with ease and grace. It's always good to reexamine and reevaluate your intentions as you move forward.

* **Make sure all of your actions are in alignment with your intention.** For instance, if you want to lose weight, don't eat donuts and cake.

* **Renew your intention regularly.** You can restate your intention every day or even multiple times a day. Then you can be sure that whatever unfolds is designed to lead you in the direction you have set. Sometimes you will have to take a circuitous route as you encounter obstacles along the way. All these things are part of the journey. Just think of it as similar to a long-distance road trip.

• • •

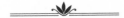

Setting a Clear Intention

1. Make sure your spine is straight. If you are sitting in a straight-backed chair, make sure your feet are on the floor. If you are sitting cross-legged on the floor, make sure your hips and buttocks are higher than your knees (sit on a blanket if necessary).

2. Close your eyes and focus on your breath as it comes in and as it goes out.

3. When you feel very relaxed, call in the light and divine love. If you wish, you can also call in your Higher Self or a spiritual master or archangel.

4. Connect to your *hara* line, the line of intention, a line of energy that runs up through your spine and down into the core of the earth. You may see the *hara* line, or visualize it, or just allow yourself to imagine it.

5. Make sure it is straight and strong. Add light to make it even brighter.

6. Contemplate what you would like to create in your life.

7. Mentally state what you desire to create. Listen to how it sounds. Is that what you want? If not, modify it until the statement rings absolutely true. To help get clarity, ask yourself why you want it.

8. State your intention in the most positive way. For instance, say, "I would like to find fulfilling work that is lucrative and fun and aligns me with my highest purpose" instead of "I would like to find work that I don't hate."

9. Fully embody the feeling of already having whatever you intend. Do this by imagining how you would feel if this goal were fulfilled. Now start feeling that way.

10. Let go of the outcome. We are not in control of how or when something comes to us.

11. When you are ready, thank the light and your Higher Self or any masters or archangels you called in. Gently come out of meditation.

12. As you go about your life, make sure all of your actions align with your intention.

13. Trust that you are being guided now. Intentions don't necessarily unfold in a linear way, and the timing is not up to us.

14. Restate your intention often, even every day or several times a day. Always connect to your hara line.

15. Notice what unfolds in your life. You may wish to use a journal.

BE PRESENT

On the surface, being present sounds easy, right? It just means really tuning in to what you are thinking and feeling. Yet our culture encourages us to do anything but tune in to our own being. We are bombarded by news; emails; texts; Facebook, Twitter, Instagram and LinkedIn posts; and all kinds of smart phone notifications. This is in addition to all the busyness of daily life with work, friends, and family. These activities and diversions give us many opportunities to be constantly tuned out.

We also have a natural tendency to want to move away from what's painful. Scarlett O'Hara declared in *Gone With the Wind*, "I'll think about that tomorrow," and that is a coping strategy many of us use. The only problem is that when you get to tomorrow, the pain is often still there.

On the other hand, if you face your pain and sit with it, it will dissolve. Your presence has a magical power. Greater peace and ease will be on the other side. Sometimes pain will momentarily intensify as we stay present with it. The pain will pass. Truly just being present, just turning around and staring at your pain or fear or anguish, will help you heal.

It's very powerful to just be present with yourself. Spend some time with yourself each day. Take a "forest bath" by going into the woods, or take a walk along the beach, or simply relax at home. Also check in with yourself regularly during the day, before you go to sleep, and when you wake up. The deep relaxation meditations on the following pages are also great for checking in, and will help you be more present the rest of the day. You will find out what's really going on, and who you are, what you want, and how you really feel. The ideal is to be present with your self in each and every moment. Try it and see.

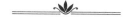

Being Present

Here is one way to be present.

1. Close yo your eyes and go deeper with each breath.

2. Allow yourself to be present with whatever is on your mind or in your heart. Just be in a state of awareness. Don't try to think about or solve anything.

3. If you have physical or emotional pain, allow it into your awareness. Don't try to move away from it.

4. As you maintain this awareness, keep focusing on your breath as you breathe in and breathe out. Allow yourself to go continually deeper. Then go even deeper.

5. When you are ready, gently come out of meditation.

Do this meditation as often as you like.

SURRENDER

Surrender is one of the most mysterious, elusive and trans-formative practices—and ultimately the most freeing. It is about trusting that whatever happens is for the best, that it is part of the process of your soul's growth. It doesn't mean that you give up, just that you accept God's will. You may keep going toward your goal, even in the face of obstacles, but offer the results to God. Everything belongs to the Divine, or if you are agnostic, the universal field.

We often think things should be different. We spend a lot of time feeling angry, sad, frustrated, despairing, resentful, discour-aged, and otherwise distressed by events and circumstances. Ironically, as soon as we surrender, we experience peace, and sometimes even ecstatic joy. Often, once we surrender, the very thing that seemed so out of reach is suddenly ours.

Surrender is not easy. I have spent years trying to surrender certain deeply held desires when they didn't seem to be in my destiny. I would think, "Finally, I surrendered," only to find I was still longing, still distressed. Instead of asking if you have truly surrendered, I suggest you ask yourself if you accept what is, with contentment and evenness of mind. Then you will know if you have surrendered.

There is a saying that an enlightened person is happy, not because he gets what he wants—but because he is happy with whatever he has. What we really want is that happiness, that contentment, that sense of fulfillment. Yet we can't just will our-selves to surrender and accept what is. It can be a deep process of self-exploration and prayer.

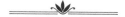

Surrender and Acceptance

For this meditation, you may want to put flowers on your altar and light a candle to create a sacred space.

1. Go into a state of deep relaxation. Close your eyes and watch your breath as it comes in and as it goes out.

2. Now see yourself entering a radiant temple. In it is an altar. There is a deity sitting on the altar. This is your own Higher Self.

3. Offer flowers to your Higher Self.

4. Thank your Higher Self for one good quality you have.

5. Thank your Higher Self for something that you have received and/or something that you wish to receive.

6. If there is something that is bothering you, such as a situation in your life or a pattern of behavior that causes you trouble, thank your Higher Self. Acknowledge the challenge as a gift for your soul's growth.

7. Thank your Higher Self for always being present for you.

8. When you are ready, you can leave the temple and, coming out of meditation, return to the present. Know that you can visit your Higher Self any time you want.

9. When you do this meditation repeatedly, you can focus on the same issue until it is resolved, or work with a variety of issues.

10. Notice what unfolds in your life.

HAVE PATIENCE

Healing should be instantaneous, right? Sometimes it is, but usually it is a process. We can have instantaneous healings and still be involved in a process that is ongoing. We can heal one pattern after another; we can erase pain grooves by making them lighter and lighter until they no longer exist. My friend Thomas Ayers, Ph.D., another healer, often talks about the glacial pace of deep transformation, and I have to agree that reshaping our inner geography takes time.

While we are healing, it sometimes may not seem as if we have accomplished much. When I worked on healing my vision, my Bates instructor told me to drop the strength of my contact lenses prescription by .50 diopters every time I had some improvement. Even though I made constant progress, my vision remained extremely blurred for a long time. I could only see dramatic results with the perspective of months and then years.

Very often there are many lessons wrapped up in one chronic challenge. For instance, I worked with a woman who had issues keeping her boundaries and not letting people push her around. She went through many tests during her healing process. With each test, her ability to stand up for herself got stronger. This is a very normal healing process.

If there is a gash in a beautiful wood floor, it will soften as soon as you begin to sand it, but it may take time before the scar is totally gone. It is the same way with deep soul grooves. These soul grooves—and we all have them—slowly soften and can ultimately fade away.

Earlier I compared a healing journey to a deep cleaning, but you could also compare it to a house renovation. Healing takes time, and things may even look more chaotic and disordered for a while along the way. That's just part of the process when you decide to knock old patterns down and create new, beautiful ways of living. Ultimately, though, you will be living in a beautiful new way and will have more ease and grace than you ever imagined.

OPEN YOUR HEART AND BE GRATEFUL

"The heart is the hub of all sacred places. Go there and roam." So said a great Indian saint, Bhagavan Nityananda. In order to access your healing power, connect to the light and love in your own heart. This light is like the sun; it shines on everyone.

The heart has a nuclear force. Through love we can resolve many different challenges, almost as if they melt away. In my experience, almost every difficulty we face, whether it is physical or situational, ultimately involves the heart. The antidote to difficulty and distress is love. Love is one of the greatest healing powers of all.

Due to the various circumstances in our lives, we don't always know exactly how to access the extraordinary force of love that is in the heart. But there is one practice that always opens the heart with ease and grace: Gratitude.

As you practice gratitude, you will experience more and more love from within and from the world outside. Be thankful for all the good things in your life. You can even be thankful for whatever pain you are experiencing, because it is there to be your teacher. If you can be grateful every day for what is occurring and truly mean it, it will change your life. Indeed, try to change your negative thoughts, as they occur, into gratitude.

You can also just picture the most beautiful, radiant light in your heart. Don't worry if you think you are imagining it; it is very real. Do this as often as you can during the day.

If there is someone with whom you want more harmony, see or imagine the light in your heart. Then experience the same light in the other person's heart. Now imagine the light of your heart and their heart connecting, even merging. Do this practice regularly, even briefly, and notice what happens.

If you are experiencing pain in some part of your body or area of your life, place the awareness of it inside this light in your heart and let it rest there. Again, do this practice regularly, and notice what happens.

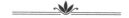

Tuning into Gratitude

1. Close your eyes and watch as your breath comes in and as it goes out.

2. Allow your mind and heart to become quieter with each breath.

3. Imagine you are entering a beautiful temple, filled with radiance.

4. As you approach the altar, see your own Higher Self sitting on the altar like a Buddha or other divine being.

5. Place your favorite flowers around the altar. You may also light candles.

6. Sit down and thank your Higher Self for one good quality you have or one good thing in your life.

7. Now thank your Higher Self for a difficulty, even your illness or pain.

8. Continue to express your gratitude for your blessings and challenges for as long as you'd like.

9. When you are ready, you can depart the temple with great respect and return to your regular space, knowing you can return as often as you wish.

RELAX DEEPLY

Relaxation is a healing state in itself, but it is undervalued in our culture. Most of the time we are dissipating our energy, but when we are relaxed, we can access our deepest wisdom and light and gather our energy.

Stress adversely affects the heart and the gut and the adrenals and sometimes other systems. It is the opposite of relaxation and is a precursor to many ills. It can lead to problems such as anxiety, acid reflux, stomach trouble, intestinal issues, heart disease, migraines and good old-fashioned exhaustion. Stress also creates disharmony in our relationships. We can't think or feel clearly when we are knotted up or feeling pressured.

Whenever I'm not feeling well, or if I experience any emotional imbalance, I take extra time for myself and go into a very deep state of relaxation, eventually slipping into a deep state of meditation as well. This type of deep relaxation slowly brings all the systems of the body—especially the heart, lungs, and nervous system—into harmony. Harmony is closely related to radiant health. When we are in a harmonious state, illnesses abate or completely resolve. Problems fade away. Simple eloquent solutions come to light.

You can use deep relaxation as a starting point for any of the guided meditations in this book. It will bring you right into the healing dimensions. Indeed, the deep relaxation journeys on the following pages are among the greatest practices you can do for yourself.

When you go into deep relaxation, you can try lying flat on your back, or you can place a very small pillow under your head. See what works best for you in terms of comfort. You can also use a blanket to keep you warm.

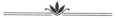

Deep Relaxation

SHORT VERSION

1. Lie on your back on a bed or on the floor. Make sure your spine is straight and that your legs are about hip-width apart. Place your hands gently at your sides with your palms up. (In hatha yoga, this pose is called *shivasana,* meaning "corpse pose." It allows your whole body to release and relax.)

2. Watch your breath as it comes in and as it goes out and let your heart and lungs fill with light.

3. Keep your attention on your breath. To make this easier, you can silently breathe in *I am the pure Self.* Then breathe out, thinking *I am totally relaxed;* or *I am radiantly healthy;* or *I love myself.*

4. Do this for as little as 10 minutes or as long as an hour or two. The longer you do it, the deeper you will go.

5. If you are very tense, don't worry, just keep returning your attention to your breath. Resist the temptation to get up. Give yourself an hour, and you will feel like a different person.

6. When you feel peaceful and are ready, gently come out of meditation.

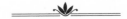

Deep Relaxation

LONG VERSION

1. Lie down on your back on a bed or the floor, with your spine straight and your legs about hip-width apart. Place your hands gently at your sides with your palms up.

2. Imagine light moving into your left foot. Allow that light to move slowly from your foot to your ankle, and then to your knee up to your hip. Feel the muscles relax as the light moves through your leg.

3. Now allow the light to move up your right foot to your ankle, and then to your knee and to your hip. Feel all the muscles relax as the light moves.

4. Let the light move through your entire lower torso and all of the organs there. Feel everything relax.

5. Now feel the light move through your abdomen, your stomach, your liver, your gallbladder, your pancreas, your kidneys in the back. Again, feel everything relax.

6. Feel the light as it fill your ribs, your heart, lungs and shoulders. Let every muscle and organ relax and fill up with light.

7. Now let the light move up through your neck and into your jaw, mouth, nose, eyes, forehead, and skull.

8. Bring your attention to the base of your spine. Imagine or feel the light move up the length of your spine and through the crown of your head.

9. Now watch your breath as it comes in and as it goes out.

10. Keep your attention on your breath. To make this easier, you can silently breathe in: *I am the pure Self.* Silently breathe out: *I am totally relaxed*; or *I am radiantly healthy*; or *I love myself.*

11. If you prefer, you can use the mantra *Ham-Sa* (pronounced "hum-sah"). Breathe in *"Hum"* and breathe out *"Sah."* Do this with every breath. The syllables have a very high vibration that will align you with universal light. (The literal translation is *"I am That."*) It is Sanskrit and the sounds resonate at the deepest levels of your being.

12. Once you are in a deep state of relaxation, you can stay there as long as you like.

13. While in this deep state, you can continue to place or imagine light everywhere in your body or specifically where you feel pain, illness or disease.

14. Gently come out of meditation when you are ready.

Do this for as little as ten minutes or as long as an hour or two. The longer you do it, the deeper you will go. If you are ill, you might do this until you feel better. Simply get up to take care of your body as you need to, and then return to deep relaxation once again.

PRAY

Prayer is an extremely powerful tool for healing. It's basically a way of opening a conversation with God—or, if you are agnostic, the universal field. Tried-and-true prayers are like a superhighway to the divine; they immediately elevate your energy.

If you have a prayer you love—whether it's a psalm or a Hail Mary, a sutra or the Sh'ma—it's a potent way to ask for help. You can start the prayer by stating your request. Then repeat the prayer as many times as you wish. You can also alternate the prayer with your request.

You can make up your own prayer, too. All you need to do is speak from your heart to God, the angels, a realized master, the four directions, your power animal, the universal field, or a nature spirit. You can pray daily, or even hourly. However you pray, it is a way to connect to God or the universal field.

When I first started to pray, I found that it was so helpful and comforting. What could be better than a conversation with God? It's a time to tell God what's going on and where you would like light, support, and guidance in your life. I pray every day; it's one way in which I stay in contact with God. I am also able to support other people because of my regular prayer practice.

You can pray before you do any of the guided meditations in this book. Your prayers will amplify your insights and the guidance you receive. Your prayers are always heard. You may not get the answer you want or get an answer in the time frame you'd like, but you will always receive help. You can ask for guidance or help with transformation, healing, understanding, acceptance and comfort.

THIRTEEN

Your Energy Anatomy

———— • • • ————

A MAP OF THE SUBTLE BODY

Your energy is the link between your body, mind and emotions, desires and intentions, and spirit. In fact, every aspect of your being is a frequency of energy. When you understand how all these different aspects of you are related, you will more fully understand yourself and your life.

Have you ever wondered how energy gets into your body? Energy moves in and around your physical body through seven major energy centers. These centers are called "chakras" from the Sanskrit word for "wheel." The first six are vortexes of energy, like whirlpools in our subtle energy, located along the spine. The first chakra is at the base of the spine. Five more energy centers are located along the spine, with a vortex at the front and back. The seventh center is at the crown of the head. Although often described as a chakra, it is an unlimited field of oneness.

The chakras modulate your energy as well as every aspect of your life. They pull in information from all around us, including from other people, and make it available for our physical, emotional, mental, and spiritual bodies.

The energy also flows up and down your central energy column, right where your spine is, connecting you to the earth and to the divine. The central column stores many of your tendencies, accumulated from how you have lived your life, and also from other incarnations.

Literally, it's all about the flow. As you'll see, each center is responsible for different areas of your body. The chakras regulate your emotional, mental, and spiritual life. The centers also direct the energy in a vast network of subtle channels that feed all of your cells, some of which are the meridians that form the basis of Chinese acupuncture. You have thousands of chakras, including at every joint, but here we will only concern ourselves with the major chakras along the spine.

The chakras are aspects of our psyche and spirit; they create our bodies and our lives. According to the Vedas, the earliest sacred texts of India, all the 50 letters of the Sanskrit alphabet—the building blocks of creation—are in the petals of the chakras. Each petal represents an energy channel that moves through that chakra and has a particular vibration that creates a subtle sound. Altogether, there are 50 channels in the first six chakras—corresponding to the 50 letters of the Sanskrit alphabet.

The chakras can be activated through these Sanskrit letters, through sound vibration and also through *bija* (seed) mantras. The *bija* or seed mantra represents the subtle sound of that particular chakra. Repeating the *bija* mantra with creative force in an enlivened way will activate the energy of that center.

The *Awakening Your Light Body System* that I teach (developed by Sanaya Roman and Duane Packer) is another way to access these energy centers in a very tangible way. The centers in this system correspond to the location of the chakras but are at a higher level of consciousness and can have a deeper, more fundamental effect. For many people, however they are easier to sense than the chakras. Three additional centers form the light body, an even more subtle and fundamental aspect of being.

When we work at these higher levels, the impact on the lower levels can be almost instantaneous. Duane Packer puts it well when he says: "If we all had equal skill levels, we'd all work at the higher levels all the time."

The more energy and dynamic flow we have in a center, the more conscious awareness we will have of the physical, emotional, mental, and spiritual issues governed by that center. When you are completely illuminated and fully conscious, your centers will be fully open, like lotuses in bloom. When you add energy to a chakra, it brings more conscious awareness; the chakra has more light and more spin; and you understand and perceive things from an expanded perspective. When these centers are spinning in a healthy fashion, the areas of the body they feed will generally be healthy. When a center is sluggish or spinning in the wrong direction, it can lead to problems.

The centers spin the way they do because of your experiences and beliefs. For instance, if you are "pissed off," that energy might clog your second chakra and cause problems in your bladder. If you are angry at God or life or a parent, you might clog the energy at your root, shutting down your basic vitality, or at your crown, so you feel disconnected from God. Everything we have explored in this book is a manifestation of how energy works.

To deepen your understanding of your energy, here's a look at each of your chakras.

YOUR SEVEN ENERGY CENTERS

FIRST CHAKRA

LOCATION:	At the base of the spine
REGULATES:	Vitality and life force, grounding, legs, feet, blood, kidneys, Roots: connection to family, ancestors, tribe
GLAND:	Adrenals
ETHERIC COLOR:	Red
BIJA MANTRA:	*Lam*

153

YOUR SEVEN ENERGY CENTERS

HOW THE CHAKRAS ALIGN IN YOUR BODY

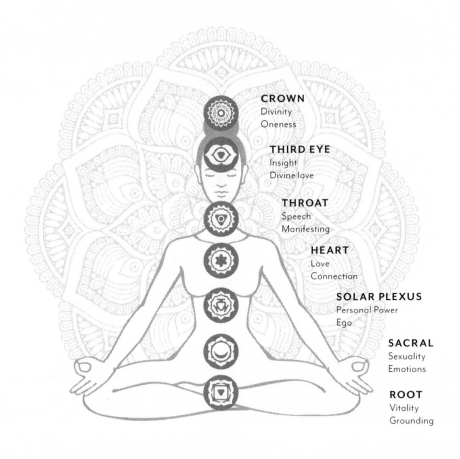

CROWN
Divinity
Oneness

THIRD EYE
Insight
Divine love

THROAT
Speech
Manifesting

HEART
Love
Connection

SOLAR PLEXUS
Personal Power
Ego

SACRAL
Sexuality
Emotions

ROOT
Vitality
Grounding

This center is sometimes called the root chakra. It is ⅃
sible for your basic vitality and life force. It also links you to y
family, ancestors, and tribe. It is what keeps you rooted and
grounded to your life here on Earth. With clairvoyant sight, it is
seen as red.

Your vitality, your "red" energy, can be enhanced through
physical exercise. Even taking a walk builds vitality, or *chi* (the
Chinese word for life force). Practices such as yoga and *tai chi* are
specifically designed to increase *chi*.

Most athletes will have a very strong and healthy first chakra.
On the other hand, someone with leukemia may lack a strong
spin in his or her first chakra. If someone's attention flits here
and there, their awareness lost in the mental plane, they could
most likely benefit from more grounding, more strength, in the
first-chakra energy (and also the third chakra, which we will get
to shortly).

When I first began investigating healing, more than a few
healers told me that I needed to be more "grounded." Initially I
had no idea what these well-intentioned healers meant. I wasn't
grounded, therefore I couldn't quite grasp the concept fully. When
we lack full consciousness in an area we also lack the ability to
fully understand that area or concept.

Eventually I realized I was living mostly in my mental body.
I had taken the world of thoughts to be the world. I needed to
be more present in my body. I could only grasp this once I was
more grounded.

Issues related to the first chakra can take all kinds of forms.
For instance, Ed came to me because of pain in his feet and toes.
When I laid hands on him, I realized the pain was, at least in
part, designed to bring his awareness back to earth—he had a
tendency to mentally fly away. I drew energy into his feet and
worked on quieting his mind and anxiety. We only worked together occasionally, but he did become more focused.

John's first-chakra issues were totally different. His father had
been abusive and his mother had lacked good boundaries. John

was damaged at the root of his being from this early trauma. He suffered from severe depression and low self-esteem. Sometimes he couldn't get out of bed. He had trouble harnessing his life force to move forward in life. In the few sessions we did together, I focused on strengthening his sense of manhood. It helped revitalize him. For a profound shift he needed healings on an ongoing basis.

The first chakra is also the home of the *Kundalini*, the spiritual energy, which in most people remains coiled in a dormant state at the base of the spine in the subtle body. When the *Kundalini* isn't awake, the subtle energy can't move up the central column towards the crown, the center of bliss and supreme consciousness. People whose *Kundalini* is asleep are therefore awake to the dream of worldly life, but asleep to the Higher Self.

When this energy is awakened, usually by initiation from a spiritual master, it begins to move up the central column, purifying all of the centers and the energies and impressions lodged in the central channel along the spine. A person's life then takes on an increasingly higher and finer vibration. Awareness and consciousness expand, along with the full flowering of potential.

The root chakra is just as important as the crown center. We need to be grounded to function at the higher levels. We need all of our energies to be complete and empowered human beings. Eventually, after the *Kundalini* is awakened and all of the centers are purified, the energy comes to rest in the crown, in supreme consciousness. That is the ultimate attainment.

Strengthening Your First (Root) Chakra
Red Energy

1. Do 20 minutes of physical exercise daily. If you want to strengthen your *chi* in a focused way, practice yoga, *Qigong*, or *Tai Chi* or study one of the martial arts, which are designed to both increase *chi* and the flow of that *chi*.

2. Make sure you are present with whatever you are doing. Are you focused on what you are doing or on the person you are with, or is your mind at the movies or on the train to Timbuktu?

3. During the day, check in with yourself to see if your mind and your actions are in the same place. If you tune in, you may be amazed—or shocked—at how busy your mind is and what a world traveler it can be.

4. Honor your ancestors, especially your mother and father. If you had a difficult relationship with your parents, find one good thing you received from each of them and inwardly appreciate and thank both of them. You can choose to focus on a different quality or experience each time you do this exercise.

5. If you wish to have your *Kundalini* energy—the dormant spiritual power that lies within everyone—awakened, you must find a true master. There is no other way to truly and completely unfold this energy. It is a very profound process of awakening and transformation. If this is your heart's desire, set your intent and keep renewing your intention. You can pray to meet an enlightened teacher, and you will be guided.

SECOND CHAKRA

LOCATION:	Below the belly button in the front and back
REGULATES:	Bladder, intestines, colon, uterus, genitals, emotions, passion, creativity, giving and receiving, boundaries
GLANDS:	Ovaries, testes
ETHERIC	Color: Orange
BIJA MANTRA:	*Vam*

The second-chakra energy guides our lives in powerful ways. It is the driving force of our passions, which evolve from our basic sexual energy combined with our emotions. Our second-chakra energy is magnetic, drawing toward us people who have similar emotional challenges, whether or not we are conscious of these challenges. This chakra also informs our decisions about the kinds of sexual energy that we respond to, and guides how we respond to that energy. Are we open and available, or are we closed off? How much emotional closeness can we accept?

Most of us treat some emotions as "good" and other emotions as "bad." Energetically, however, what's most important is to let your emotions move through you the way clouds move through the sky. Whether you feel sadness, loneliness, anger, bitterness, passion, or joy, you don't want to either repress your emotions or to let them drive you. You also don't want to wallow in them. The key words are "flow" and "detachment."

When you hold in your emotions or let yourself drown in them, it affects the flow of energy through the rest of the body. Whatever emotional issues you don't process will prevent you from thinking, seeing, and acting clearly. The same is true for your sexual energy. You want it to flow in a way that doesn't control you without your conscious awareness.

When you can't process emotions and allow them to flow, you can end up with digestive issues, bladder infections, and depression. A person with colitis may have a second chakra that is sluggish or even spinning backward.

A sluggish second chakra can also affect a person's ability to give and receive—it can lead to constipation at the physical level. If there is a general energy of withholding, then a person can begin to heal by consciously giving on material, emotional, and spiritual levels.

Sexual and reproductive issues can also be linked to this chakra. A man who can't deeply connect emotionally or who lacks self-confidence may experience premature or quick ejaculation; he may be unwilling to engage sexually at all.

A woman who doesn't have strong boundaries may leave herself open to receiving unwanted sexual energy from others. It may seem as if she is receiving a lot of attention when in fact she is draining herself of her own power. This transaction, which is not truly conscious, can lead to ill health in her reproductive organs.

Many people need a great deal of support to develop good emotional flow and clear boundaries.

Strengthening Your Second (Pelvic) Chakra
Orange Energy

1. Allow yourself to be aware of your feelings. Difficult emotions are perfectly fine as long as you resolve them. Let them flow through you instead of trying to hold them down.

2. Treat your sexuality and sexual organs with dignity, respect, and honor.

3. Create appropriate boundaries. Don't let people push you around or make you do something you do not want to do.

4. Practice healthy giving and receiving of both emotional and sexual energies in your relationships.

5. Notice to whom you are sexually attracted. Try to understand that person's qualities and notice where these qualities exist in you. If they are qualities you like, enhance them. If they are qualities you don't like, work on dissolving these issues in yourself.

6. Understand and always respect the sacred nature of your passions, both sexual and creative. For instance, sex shouldn't be treated as a sporting activity, but rather as the expression of a sacred bond. You can even pray or meditate together before intimate union.

THIRD CHAKRA

LOCATION:	Solar plexus, in the front and back of the body.
REGULATES:	Stomach, liver, gallbladder, kidneys, spleen, personal will, ego, intellect, relationship cords
GLAND:	Pancreas
ETHERIC COLOR:	Yellow
BIJA MANTRA:	*Ram*

The third chakra is located in the solar plexus, above the navel, in the hollow below the rib cage. On the physical level, this center regulates the digestive fire and the major abdominal organs including the pancreas, liver, gallbladder, and stomach. On the emotional level, the third chakra is a key location for the energy cords that connect you to others with whom you have relationships.

This is your power center. Much of your ego, intellect, and personal will is centered in the third chakra. Possessiveness, fear, shame, anxiety, and anger can reside in this chakra and potentially disturb the well-being of your organs. When your relationships are tangled, it will often show up in your gut. When there is anxiety, it can cause a contraction that makes it difficult for energy to flow up into the heart, creating a feeling of disconnection and loneliness.

There is a profound solar radiance that occurs in this chakra when you clear it of tangles, but we are, by and large, a third-chakra nation. As a society, we tend to emphasize the intellect over the heart. Anxiety, fear, anger, and control are major causes of contraction at this chakra. Knots in this center can also cause difficulties in relationships. I've softened and dissolved more than a few third-chakra knots.

People who don't want to experience their emotions will often use the third chakra to keep that information from rising up through the chakras and into consciousness. They may eat too much to keep the emotions down, or they may develop various other types of desires or addictions (attachments) in an effort to appease various feelings such as loneliness, unworthiness, or a deep, nameless hunger for love. Of course, if we could let all of that energy flow into our hearts, we'd feel much better—and be less attached and needy.

This chakra is the central location for the feeling of "doership"—the belief that you must take care of everything or the world will fall down. And when you contract the energy of this chakra through your desires and longings, thoughts and fears, ambitions and will, judgment and anger, you may also contract the energy that can move up into the heart.

The unresolved energies of the third chakra can drive a person to great heights. However, there is no peace until you begin to clear the various issues and desires clogging this chakra. When you let the energy flow, it moves into the heart, and you experience fulfillment.

Strengthening Your Third (Solar Plexus) Chakra
Yellow Energy

1. Try to keep your relationships free and clear of entanglements. Avoid doing anything because you expect someone to do something for you. When you give, give freely.

2. Start to notice your addictions. For instance, if you eat too much, pause when you've eaten a little less than usual. Give yourself 20 minutes and see how you feel. What comes up if you don't stuff yourself? If you are addicted to a relationship, see how you feel when you can't be with that person.

3. Try to accept things as they are instead of trying to control everything.

4. Transmute tendencies such as anger, jealousy, worry, fear, and mental agitation. You can do this through meditation, prayer, and other spiritual practices.

5. Eat a balanced diet. Be careful not to eat an excess of sugar or simple carbohydrates, which will adversely affect your mood, your mental state, and the health of your body. While sugars give you a quick lift, they ultimately leave you feeling depleted and empty.

6. Eat moderate amounts. When you eat too much, a lot of energy is taken up by digestion, making you sluggish and leaving less energy for projects, activities, and relationships.

FOURTH CHAKRA

LOCATION:	At the sternum, front and back
REGULATES:	Heart, lungs, chest, love, inner peace, spiritual connection, seat of the individual soul
GLAND:	Thymus
ETHERIC COLOR:	Green
BIJA MANTRA:	*Yam*

The fourth chakra, also known as the heart chakra, is in the center of our chest. This chakra is at the very center of our energy body, located between the three lower centers and the three upper centers, bridging our personality and soul. You could think of it as the sacred space where Heaven and Earth unite.

In Eastern traditions, the heart is known as the seat of the soul. In Chinese medicine, the heart is considered the seat of the mind. This is the view of the Vedic scriptures from India as well: When the heart is at peace, so is the mind. In Christian teachings, Jesus is often depicted with a flaming heart, the great Heart of Oneness. In the Kabbalah, the heart energies of Tijeret—balance and harmony—are at the very center of the Tree of Life. The energy of the heart is a nuclear force: If you give it time to do its magic, it can melt almost any pain, but this requires staying present. Sometimes the pain can seem so overwhelming that we feel we have to do something or move away or distract ourselves, and yet if we just stay with the pain, it will release.

At the center of the spiritual journey is the purification of the individual heart so we can merge into the Supreme Heart of oneness. Some of the difficult energies that we encounter in the heart are anxiety, arrogance, indecision, and regret, but all of these can be transmuted. Hope, endeavor, and discernment are positive attributes that reside in this center.

You can understand a lot about a person's heart chakra just by getting to know him or her. Is this person accepting? Kind? Generous? Judgmental?

Almost all illness involves a withdrawal of love in one form or another, and thus many different illnesses have a link with the heart chakra. If you can fully love and accept whatever is going on, you can heal a great deal.

Medical studies show that many different illnesses affect the energy of the heart. Anxiety, for instance, will cause the heart energy to be very agitated. Depression, alcoholism, diabetes, and many other diseases are all linked to low heart rate variability, an electromagnetic energy pattern in which the heart rhythm lacks an exuberant range.

When we reach a state of inner peace, we can connect to others heart to heart. When we completely purify our heart we experience the radiant bliss of our Supreme Heart, a state of oneness. This is the ultimate goal of our spiritual journey. As I mention in Chapter 12: "Seven Essentials for Healing," a great Indian master once said: "The heart is the hub of all sacred places. Go there and roam."

Strengthening Your Fourth (Heart) Chakra
Green Energy

1. Practice forgiveness and cultivate qualities such as trust, faith, gratitude, and acceptance. These qualities will transform your life and your heart.

2. Offer selfless service—for example, tutor a child or volunteer at a soup kitchen. Serving others in a selfless way, without the expectation of receiving anything in return, opens the heart and lets its exquisite light shine.

3. Pray and/or meditate. Both of these practices are like gymnastics for the heart and will help make your heart more supple. Meditation helps bring your mind to rest in your heart. This creates an expanded heart rhythm that allows you to feel peaceful and experience harmony in your life. It also brings your heart, breath, and brain waves into resonance with one another, creating better health.

FIFTH CHAKRA

LOCATION:	Throat, front and back
REGULATES:	Throat, ears (with the sixth chakra), vocal cords, speaking, listening, hearing, manifesting, aspects of giving and receiving, living your dream

GLAND: Thyroid

ETHERIC COLOR: Blue

BIJA MANTRA: *Ham*

Flow in the fifth chakra is critical for creating what we want in the world. Located at the throat, this center feeds energy to the throat, thyroid, mouth, neck, and ears. It regulates speaking and hearing, creativity and manifesting. A flow in this center helps us manifest and live our dreams. The Word, of course, is intimately connected to creation. At the very beginning of the Bible, God's first act of creation is through the Word: "God said, Let there be light: and there was light." In both the Kabbalah and Sanskrit texts, there is something known as the power of the alphabet—what is known in Sanskrit as matrika shakti. The words we use, the thoughts we think, are powerful creative forces—more powerful than most of us can imagine. The Zohar, the mystical text of the Old Testament, teaches that the energies of the alphabet were manifest before the creation of the world.

Speaking the truth and speaking from your heart are practices that support flow in this chakra. When we can't speak up, it can be difficult to create what we want. I had a lot of issues in my fifth chakra when I first began to explore my own energy—for example, although I could express my thoughts, it was hard for me to speak from my heart if I was afraid that someone would be angry with me.

You can usually hear what someone is feeling in his or her voice. If someone's voice is tight, that person is probably tense. If it is quivering, he or she is emotional. When we speak from our hearts, our words have great resonance. It is equally important to be able to listen to others with your heart.

The fifth chakra is also involved with timing, with the rhythms of the body and with knowing when to speak and when not to speak. It is with the energies in this chakra that we can begin to hear and obey our Higher Self. Spiritually, it is at this level of light that our true and perfect template, sometimes known as the etheric template, exists. When we are "true blue," it means we are in integrity. When we are "feeling blue," however, it may be because we are not manifesting our dreams or living in our truth.

There are 16 petals in the throat chakra. Each one has a different quality. One petal, for example, has the energy of venom. With another petal you tap the energy of nectar. We can always choose what we want to convey when we speak, and I recommend focusing on nectar.

You can have a sense of what is going on in someone's throat chakra by noticing whether that person speaks up or not. Does he or she speak the truth? And listen carefully? Someone who cannot listen to others or is not heard by others obviously has some blockage in the energy in this center. When a person uses his or her voice to force his will, it can lead to a hyperthyroid condition. A person who has difficulty expressing his or her heart's truth or creativity may eventually develop a low-functioning thyroid.

There are always resonances between the second and fifth chakras. For instance, if a person has a lot of sexual shame or repression, there may be blocks in both the second and fifth chakras.

Physical issues involving the throat or neck generally indicate an imbalance in the fifth chakra. The cervical discs, located in the neck, may also give us clues to issues in other energy centers, as well. For instance, someone who has an injury between the fourth and fifth cervical discs in the neck may be having difficulty speaking from his or her heart.

Strengthening Your Fifth (Throat) Chakra
Blue Energy

1. Always speak the truth. This empowers your words and supports your ability to create and manifest. It honors the power of the Word.

2. Listen to others with the same respect you would like to receive when you are speaking.

3. Learn to speak up when appropriate. Also know when to observe silence.

4. Chanting and singing can strengthen this chakra. So can writing, painting, and other forms of self-expression.

5. Follow God's will. Listen to your inner voice.

6. Pursue your dreams, but only by performing right action—in other words, live by the Golden Rule.

SIXTH CHAKRA

LOCATION:	Between the eyebrows, front and back of the head
REGULATES:	Vision and eyes (with the third chakra), insight, intuition, creativity, clairvoyance, divine love, detachment, Gland: Pineal & Pituitary
ETHERIC COLOR:	Violet
BIJA MANTRA:	*Om*

This chakra oversees insight, intuition, vision, creativity and clairvoyance. It is the seat of the mystical third eye. The sixth chakra also regulates our sense of faith and our experience of divine love. Generally, our third eye can work most optimally when we clear the energies in the other chakras. People who have a tendency to get headaches may be contracting energy in this region because they are afraid to see or look too closely at something in their lives.

Of course, most of us have blind spots. These begin with the way we run our energy in the first, second, and third chakras. We need the life force energy from the first chakra for healthy eyes. We need to clear emotional issues from the second chakra to see emotional patterns clearly. For example, if you had a parent who suffered from depression and you were unaware of their depression, you might draw depressed people into your inner sphere.

I used to joke that I had a cataract over my third eye. I wouldn't allow myself to see people clearly when I had some personal investment in seeing only their good qualities. It was extremely painful. Actually, I did see clearly, but I didn't trust my vision. It took a great deal of healing work and focused intention to begin to clear this chakra and trust my inner vision.

Strengthening Your Sixth (Third Eye) Chakra Violet Energy

1. Prayer, meditation, and spiritual practice can support your vision and your faith.

2. Selfless service—service done without an attachment to receiving benefit or gain—will support this chakra (and, indeed, all of your chakras).

3. Honor and act upon your vision, and your vision will grow more clear.

4. See through the eyes of love and the eye of the heart.

THE SEVENTH CHAKRA:
THE CROWN

LOCATION: Crown of the head

REGULATES: Direct connection to the Divine One-
                    ness, union with God

ETHERIC COLOR: White

GLAND: Pituitary, along with the sixth center

The seventh center, also known as the crown center, is at the top of the head. It has the most exquisite white light. The Sanskrit alphabet repeats itself twenty times in this center, creating a thousand petals of scintillating brilliance. Our divine light emanates from here. This is the center of supreme consciousness.

Attaining this light is the ultimate goal of human life. Halos are often depicted in paintings above the heads of saints. This is to show that they are illuminated by their conscious connection to the divine through the crown chakra. I often see beautiful bright light around people who do spiritual practices such as prayer, selfless service, and meditation. Before we can attain the full fruits of this level of light, we must surrender fully to the will of God.

Strengthening Your Connection to Your Seventh Center
Radiant White Energy

1. Hold the intention to be aligned with God's will.

2. Meditate.

3. Cultivate spiritual practices.

4. Serve others with selfless love.

A Final Note About Chakras

The chakras function in relation to one another. You can think of each chakra as a color of the rainbow or a note on a musical scale—in fact, at the level of the emotional body, the chakras make a rainbow of color, and each chakra has its own tone. Every one of us is a walking rainbow and a symphony of energies.

The energies from the chakras can be combined in infinite ways, with infinite effects. Our chakras are always interacting, and each cell in our body is bathed in the energy from all seven chakras. Most physical, emotional and spiritual issues, I find, aren't truly confined to just one chakra.

Please remember, too, that the chakras are only the beginning of the story. They are just one dimension more subtle than the physical world. In reality, our subtle body extends into far more subtle, or causal, levels. Energies such as harmony, gentleness, faith, trust and grace can have a positive, global effect on your energy system.

With this map of your energy anatomy, you can begin to understand yourself in a much deeper way. For instance, if you notice that you have a lot of tension in your gut, you may want to contemplate what might be going on in your relationships or attachments. Beginning to heal on that level may alleviate your physical symptoms. If you are feeling blue, you might ask yourself, Am I living my dream? How can I start to make my dreams a reality?

Perhaps you notice that you are drawn to wearing orange or even eating orange foods—you just love orange. This may mean you need more orange power, more orange energy. For instance, I had a client who was scheduled for a hysterectomy. In the weeks before and following the surgery, she always instinctively wore orange when she came to see me. She had no idea of the relationship between energy centers and color frequencies. However, the womb is just behind the second chakra, which radiates an orange frequency. She wore orange because she needed energy support in that area.

When I was healing both my physical vision and my relationship to my inner vision, I gravitated toward violets and purples, the color of the sixth chakra. I had purple clothes, purple curtains in my bedroom, purple towels, purple dining chairs, and a purple prayer shawl. I even had lavender-colored luggage. You name it, it was a shade of purple. I couldn't get enough purple.

Years earlier, I painted my living room walls blue with white trim. This was a time when my fifth chakra, or throat chakra, was in great distress. I didn't know consciously back then that I had emotional blockages in this center that made me afraid to fully speak my truth. I didn't even know anything about chakra energies and colors when I did this painting. When I finally repainted everything white (with a subtle pink wash over it), I felt as if I had been released from prison. I had done healings to clear my throat center, and the blue color on the wall had become oppressive.

All that said, I doubt color treatment alone, even on an ongoing basis, would completely reset one's chakras. These things take time, and they are usually very deep. It is best to work with subtle energy to transmute energies at the subtle level. I am merely noting the relationship between colors and chakras to give you a diagnostic tool.

The chakras are a key to understanding yourself. The chakras can give you insight into your emotional and mental patterns and how they interact with your physical body.

YOUR CHAKRA SYSTEM

Chakra	Location	Regulates	Gland
First	Base of Spine	Vitality and life force. Legs, feet, blood, kidneys. Grounding and connection to family, ancestors and tribe. Sense of smell.	Adrenals
Second	Below the belly button	Bladder, intestines, colon, uterus, genitals. Emotions, passion, creativity. Giving and receiving. Boundaries; Sense of taste.	Ovaries, Testes
Third	Solar Plexus	Stomach, liver, gallbladder, pancreas, spleen, kidneys (with first chakra). Personal will, ego, intellect. Relationship cords. Sense of sight.	Pancreas
Fourth	Heart	Heart, lungs, chest. Love, inner peace, spiritual connection. Seat of the individual soul. Sense of touch.	Thymus
Fifth	Throat	Throat, ears (with the sixth chakra), vocal cords. Speaking and listening. Manifesting. Aspects of giving and receiving. Living your dream. Sense of hearing.	Thyroid
Sixth	In the center of the head, between the eyebrows.	Eyes (with 3rd chakra). Inner vision, insight, clairvoyance, intuition, creativity. Divine love.	Pineal/ Pituitary
Seventh	Crown of the Head	Direct connection to the Divine. Oneness.	Pituitary

THE CHAKRAS AND THEIR POWERS

Chakra	*Bija* Mantra	Associated Element	Associated Sense Perception	Associated Power of Action
1	*Lam*	Earth	Smell	Locomotion
2	*Vam*	Water	Taste	Grasping
3	*Ram*	Fire	Sight	Excretion
4	*Yam*	Air	Touch	Reproduction
5	*Ham*	Ether	Hearing	Speaking
6	*Om*	Mind/Primordial Nature	Mind	Mind
7	Subtle Impressions left by *Om*	Supreme Consciousness	Supreme Consciousness	Supreme Consciousness

FOURTEEN

Body Symbology

— • • • —

The information in the Body Symbology chart below is just a taste of the infinite ways in which our souls speak to us through our bodies. I've been doing healings for many years, and I still find that each healing is a revelation because each one of us is unique. The examples below are generalizations. But the chart can be a very useful guide to begin to go deeper within your self.

Body Area/Issue	Underlying Issue or Theme
Acid reflux	Something in your life may be hard to swallow, something in your past may be coming up for resolution.
Anxiety	Involves in an inability to connect to or trust your Inner Self and the process of life, often due to childhood emotional trauma. It can also be absorbed from anxious parents.
Addictions	Seeking something outside one's self to fill a lack or cover over insecurity, low self-esteem, or other difficult feelings. An inability to connect inwardly/to spirit for comfort and connection.

Body Area/Issue	Underlying Issue or Theme
Arrhythmia	May indicate a desire for a more open heart/spiritual awareness.
Arteries, blockages in	Might be related to ways you've closed down your emotional/spiritual heart.
Back	Feeling supported. See "Your Energy Anatomy" as well. In the sacrum or behind the solar plexus it might be related to a relationship issue. In the area behind the heart it might be connected to strengthening self love.
Bladder	Are you "pissed off"?
Blood pressure, high	Deep-seated anger, fear or frustration; pressure to perform may be bottled up.
Cancer	A part of you wants more freedom or empowerment. Can involve feelings of frustration or despair about a life situation. More nuanced meaning is generally related to the location in your body. A cancer in the breast may have a different meaning than a cancer involving the optic nerve or a cancer in the throat.
Chronic fatigue	Past trauma or feelings of not being worthy may be driving you to exhaustion.
Depression	Anger turned inward; Not living fully; Not believing you have the power you need in life. Lack of spiritual connection.
Diabetes	Are you taking in the sweetness of life?
Disturbance to the face (e.g.. Bell's palsy)	May reflect that there is something you are having difficulty facing.
Ears	Involves hearing or listening.

Body Area/Issue	Underlying Issue or Theme
Eyes	Issues with seeing and knowing.
Feet	Being grounded; standing in your power.
Gallbladder	Decision-making and mental clarity; having the nerve and courage to act.
Genitals	Masculine and feminine energies.
Hands	What you can handle, hold.
Heart	A call to experience more love, enthusiasm, joy; connection to spirit; embracing yourself, others.
Hips	May indicate a need to work on better connection in your romantic relationship.
Hyperthyroidism	May be related to ways in which you are trying too hard.
Hypothyroidism	May be connected to difficulty in speaking up or expressing your creativity.
Infections (bacterial)	May be fueled by unresolved emotion, such as anger.
Infections (viral)	May indicate that a life pattern or belief needs to be reexamined and transformed.
Intestines	May involve difficulty digesting emotions or setting boundaries.
Irritable Bowel Syndrome	May be related to unresolved emotional irritations. What is irritating you?
Kidneys	Where fear is processed and stored.

Body Area/Issue	Underlying Issue or Theme
Left Side of the Body	May indicate you need to resolve something about your feminine energies or a relationship with a woman/women in your life.
Legs	Moving forward, standing in your power; sometimes issues here stem from not feeling supported by someone in your life.
Liver	Where anger and physical toxins are processed and stored.
Lungs	Sadness and grief.
Neck/Throat	May be an invitation to learn to speak up, speak the truth. Issues here can also be caused by words having been used to assault you. Living your dream.
Right Side of the Body	May suggest you need to resolve something about your masculine energies or a relationship with a man/men in your life.
Sexually Transmitted Disease	Could be an invitation to strengthen your boundaries/ sense of self. Sexual shame.
Shoulders	Burdens you don't need to carry. What are the "should-ers" you are taking on?
Pancreas	The place in the body where sweetness is processed. (See diabetes)
Stomach	Digesting food and ideas; worry; what's eating you?
Uterus	Feminine power; creativity.

Body Area/Issue	Underlying Issue or Theme
Weight, Excess	Can be a protection resulting from sexual or emotional trauma or having one's boundaries violated. It may also be caused by low self-esteem. An inability to fully engage and move forward in your life. Being oversensitive, needing protection. Holding anger and resentment. What is weighing you down?

FIFTEEN

As You Continue Your Journey

———— · ● · ————

Blessings to you for radiant health and joy. Follow your inner guidance. Know that the light is always there to protect, help and guide you. You can ask for help from your Higher Self, the masters, saints, angels or other higher beings. No request is too large or too small. If you want help, you must ask. As Jesus himself taught, if you ask, you shall receive. The ascended masters will always come to your aid, whether you can perceive it or not. Always remember that you are a divine being, a child of God.

Acknowledgments

————— • • • —————

I'm grateful to you, dear reader, for taking the time to read this book. I'm grateful, too, for all of you who have come for healings or to study energy healing with me and thus share light; and to my teachers—in particular, Rosalyn Bruyere, Barbara Brennan, Amy Skezas, Jason Shulman, Sanaya Roman and Duane Packer, Gerda Swearengen, Thomas C. Ayers, Ph.D., and Dianne Arnold, for your wisdom, healing light and compassion. A special thanks also to Gerda and Thomas for always being there, especially in the early years.

Endless gratitude to my dear parents, Roslyn and Howard Goldner, my first teachers, who have always offered thoughtfulness, love and support. A special thanks and love to my husband, Mike, and my son, Max. You've opened a sacred world of love.

Thanks also to my many dear friends and companions on the spiritual path. I especially want to acknowledge Lars and JoAnn Svanberg, hosts for so many years on my visits to the East End of Long Island, and to Sonam Kushner, Ellen Sackoff and Rick Aidekman, Susan McArdle, Jolie Parcher and Robert Abramson, M.D., for sharing their beautiful healing spaces with me during my many trips to New York.

A special acknowledgement to Laurie Campbell, Lorrie Kazan and Allison DuBois, who, over the years, have sent so many wonderful people to me for healings. I also want to acknowledge my friends and fellow light-workers: energy healer Nancy Reuben, M.D.; healer and energy tracker Judy Eggleston; tarot reader Susan Kim; and clairvoyant guide Karen Campbell—a special thanks for all your help and support in the writing and publishing process.

Thank you to my friend and former magazine colleague Jenny Cook for your editing and to Amy Gingery for such an inspired and beautiful book design, and for being so in tune. My gratitude to Robert Kemter for reading this manuscript on so many levels, and sharing so much illumination and insight. I know you were sent by the Masters. My gratitude to Robert Boress, sent by the angels to offer guidance, editing, and final proofing just when I needed it.

A special thanks to Lynn Falkowski for reading and commenting on the manuscript; to Tracy Raynor, JoAnn Svanberg, Susan Vroom, healers Dani Antman and Adriana Barone, and bestselling authors Karen Page and Andrew Dornenburg for cover inspiration and guidance.

My unending gratitude to the Spiritual Master who woke me up and guides me every step of the way. Her love and support and grace is what makes all of this possible.

About the Author

—— • • • ——

D iane Goldner is an internationally known healer. She helps people facing physical, emotional and spiritual challenges involving illness, injury and infertility, and works with people to resolve life issues involving money, relationships, boundaries, self-esteem and personal transformation.

A *cum laude* graduate of Barnard College and a journalist, Diane began investigating healing as a skeptic. After discovering that healing could have powerful results, a five-year investigation led to her first book, *How People Heal,* published in hardcover as *Infinite Grace: Where the Worlds of Science and Spiritual Healing Meet.*

During this period she was mentored by some of the most gifted healers teaching at that time, and began her studies with a realized master from India, versed in the *Vedas* and other sacred texts. She describes the profound process of becoming a healer in her second book, *Awakening to the Light,* a memoir of spiritual awakening.

Diane does hands-on healing in Los Angeles, Manhattan and the Hamptons, and long-distance healing with people across the United States and in other countries. She also teaches healing and subtle energy skills on both coasts and via webinars. She is a recommended resource in Christine Northrup, M.D.'s *New York*

Times bestseller, *Women's Bodies, Women's Wisdom*. Diane has discussed healing on dozens of radio and television programs including CNN and Hay House Radio, and has given talks at Canyon Ranch, the University of Arizona Medical School, Children's Memorial Hospital in Chicago, and at healing centers and bookstores. She was the Healer in Residence at the Cornelia Spa in New York City during its Guest Expert Program.

As a former journalist, Diane has written for *The New York Times, The Wall Street Journal, American Health, Health, Healthy Living,* and many other publications. She served as senior editor at *Fame* and as a contributing editor at *Variety* and at *USA Weekend,* where she wrote cover stories and launched and edited a summer fiction series featuring bestselling authors. Diane got her start as an investigative journalist for *The American Lawyer*. She has written about healing for Beliefnet.com, Money.com and other publications.

Diane lives with her husband and son in Los Angeles, California, and travels regularly to NYC and the Hamptons to teach and give healings.

To learn more, download guided meditations, sign up for Diane's monthly e-newsletter or find a workshop, go to www. DianeGoldner.com. You can also e-mail Diane at DianeGoldner@ gmail.com.

To arrange for group orders, or to book Diane to speak to your group, healing circle or at your event, please e-mail Diane at DianeGoldner@gmail.com.

Awakening to the Light

(First published as *A Call to Heal*)

———— • • • ————

"I Love this book. It's wonderful. And so inspiring."

—CHRISTIANE NORTHRUP, M.D., author of the *New York Times* bestseller *Women's Bodies, Women's Wisdom*

"Awakening to the Light is an absolute gem. Diane has written an amazing account of a life turned upside down in the most beautiful way. This is a must read for anyone seeking a deeper connection with a more profound meaning and direction in life."

—JULIE HOYLE, author of *An Awakened Life*

"Can a book heal? This one does. It has an energy that is released to the reader. I felt it. As a healer myself, I could relate to everything Diane so candidly describes. If you read only one book on healing make it this one. This book should be a movie."

—SUSAN MCARDLE, Executive Director,
Joshua's Place Healing Center

"I could not put this book down once I began reading. Diane's gift for writing allows you to relate to her journey in a very personal way. The book gave me goose bumps many times. It has become my favorite, which I now keep beside my bed, and flick to a page for wisdom, comfort, inspiration or peace."

—RE HAYNES, Australia

"After I finished reading, I lay down and closed my eyes. The angels came and you were there. I had a healing of a pain that had been bothering me for years."

—KAREN FLYNN, clairvoyant

How People Heal

—— • • • ——

"I love *How People Heal*. Diane has done society a good deed with this book."

—MEHMET OZ, M.D., author of *Healing from the Heart* and host of *"The Dr. Oz Show"*

"*How People Heal* is absolutely wonderful. Reading it gave me the chills and filled me with hope, awe, and gratitude. It's a road map to the unknown and unrecognized power within us all."

—CHRISTIANE NORTHRUP, M.D., author of *The New York Times* bestseller *Women's Bodies, Women's Wisdom*

"Wisdom and vision, page after page."

—GARY SCHWARTZ, PHD, and Linda Russek, authors of *The Living Energy Universe*

"This work is particularly inspired. Reading it I felt I was actually embraced with Grace. I have a feeling that Diane Goldner has really been sent to us as a messenger."

—NICHOLAS CIMORELLI, host of *"Health Action,"* WBAI-NY

"Credible and thought-provoking, this book is a must-read for anyone aspiring to be an energy healer or considering energy healing as a therapy."

—NATURAL HEALTH